D1321880

# Intercollegiate MRCS: EMQ Practice Papers

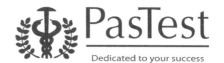

PasTest

Dedicated to your success

# Intercollegiate MRCS: EMQ Practice Papers

**Kimberly Lammin**
BSc MBChB MRCS
Specialist Registrar,
Trauma and Orthopaedics,
Royal Preston Hospital

**Lorna Cook**
BA MBBS MRCS
Clinical Fellow in General Surgery
Royal Sussex County Hospital, Brighton

**Amol Chitre**
MBChB MRCS (England)
Senior SHO
Trauma and Orthopaedics
Royal Bolton Hospital

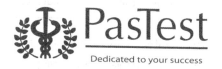

PasTest
Dedicated to your success

© 2006 PASTEST LTD

Egerton Court
Parkgate Estate
Knutsford
Cheshire
WA16 8DX

Telephone: 01565 752000

First published 2006

ISBN: 1 904627 978
ISBN: 978 1 904627 975

A catalogue record for this book is available from the British Library.

**PasTest Revision Books and Intensive Courses**

*PasTest has been established in the field of postgraduate medical education since 1972, providing revision books and intensive study courses for doctors preparing for their professional examinations.*

Books and courses are available for the following specialties:

MRCGP, MRCP Parts 1 and 2, MRCPCH Parts 1 and 2, MRCPsych, MRCS, MRCOG Parts 1 and 2, DRCOG, DCH, FRCA, PLAB Parts 1 and 2, Dental Students, Dentists and Dental Nurses.

For further details contact:

**PasTest, Freepost, Knutsford, Cheshire WA16 7BR**

**Tel: 01565 752000**          **Fax: 01565 650264**

**www.pastest.co.uk**          **enquiries@pastest.co.uk**

Text prepared by Carnegie Book Production, Lancaster

Printed and bound in Great Britain by Antony Rowe Ltd, Chippenham, Wiltshire

# Contents

# Foreword

This book is aimed at MRCS candidates and contains 3 complete practice papers each consisting of 180 questions.

The book was written by people who recently sat the examination with the aim of providing papers similar to those being used currently. Each paper covers the same variety of topics as laid out in the intercollegiate MRCS syllabus and the questions are of varying degrees of difficulty, in order to make the papers as similar to the exam as possible. Several topics are covered in more than one paper, reflecting the fact that these are frequently asked about.

The questions consist of a topic followed by a list of options and then the questions that are linked to that stem. Each answer can be used once, not at all or more than once.

The book aims to provide candidates with valuable practice at extended matching questions in advance of the exam, and to aid candidates in identifying areas of weakness for further study. It is designed to be used in conjunction with the recommended MRCS textbooks, and does not cover every topic.

We hope you will find this book useful.

Good Luck

Kim and Amol

# Examination technique

This is a brief guide which we hope you will find helpful for the EMQ paper of the MRCS.

Most of the points mentioned below are fairly obvious, but during the stress of the exam it is easy to forget some of them.

**Revision**

- Start revising early, you never have as much time as you think you do.
- Try to revise with someone else sitting the same exam
- Do plenty of practice questions so that you are familiar with the format

**In the exam itself**

- Read the instructions carefully
- Allow enough time to complete the paper
- If you are initially writing the answers on the questions sheet, make sure you allow time to transfer them to the answer sheet
- Always turn over the last page, you wouldn't be the first person to miss the last few questions
- Read the questions thoroughly
- If the question seems too simple, it probably *is* that straightforward; there should not be any trick questions in the exam.

Good luck.

# Abbreviations

| | |
|---|---|
| A&E | Accident and Emergency |
| AAA | abdominal aortic aneurysm |
| ABPI | ankle–brachial pressure index |
| ACL | anterior cruciate ligament |
| ACTH | adrenocorticotropic hormone |
| AIN | anal intra-epithelial neoplasis |
| AP | anteroposterior |
| ASA | American Society of Anesthesiologists |
| ASB | assisted spontaneous breathing |
| BCG | bacille Calmette-Guérin |
| BIPAP | biphasic positive airway pressure |
| BMI | body mass index |
| BPH | benign prostatic hyperplasia |
| CEA | carcinoembryonic antigen |
| CIS | carcinoma in situ |
| CMV | continuous mandatory ventilation |
| CPAP | continuous positive airway pressure |
| CRP | C-reactive protein |
| CT | computed tomography |
| CVP | central venous pressure |
| DDH | developmental dysplasia of the hip |
| DRE | digital rectal examination |
| ECG | electrocardiogram |
| ESR | erythrocyte sedimentation rate |
| ESWL | extracorporal shock wave lithotripsy |
| FBC | full blood count |
| GCS | Glasgow Coma Scale |

| | |
|---|---|
| GGT | $\gamma$-glutamyl transferase |
| GTN | glyceryl trinitrate |
| hCG | human chorionic gonadotrophin |
| HIV | human immunodeficiency virus |
| ICU | intensive care unit |
| IVU | intravenous urogram |
| KUB | kidney-ureter-bladder (X-ray) |
| MEN | multiple endocrine dysplasia |
| NPV | negative predictive value |
| NSAID | non-steroidal anti–inflammatory drug |
| PCNL | percutaneous nephrolithotomy |
| PDS | polydioxanone suture |
| PEG | percutaneous endoscopic gastrostomy |
| PPV | positive predictive value |
| PSA | prostate-specific antigen |
| PTH | parathyroid hormone |
| RIF | right iliac fossa |
| RTA | road traffic accident |
| RUQ | right upper quadrant |
| SIMV | synchronous intermittent mandatory ventilation |
| SLE | systemic lupus erythematosus |
| SUFE | slipped upper femoral epiphysis |
| TPN | total parenteral nutrition |
| TURBT | transurethral resection of bladder tumour |
| TURP | transurethral resection of prostate |
| TWOC | trial without catheter |
| U&E | urea and electrolytes |
| UTI | urinary tract infections |
| VMA | vanillylmandelic acid |

# QUESTIONS

# QUESTIONS
# PRACTICE PAPER 1

## THEME: TREATMENT OF TESTICULAR TUMOURS

**A**  Chemotherapy

**B**  Chemotherapy and radiotherapy

**C**  Orchidectomy and prophylactic radiotherapy

**D**  Orchidectomy and surveillance

**E**  Radiotherapy

**F**  Retroperitoneal lymph node dissection

**G**  Testicular biopsy

For each of the following scenarios, choose the most appropriate treatment from the list above. Each option may be used once, more than once or not at all.

1  A 22-year-old man presents with hard swelling of left testis and undergoes orchidectomy. Histological examination shows non-seminomatous germ cell tumour. Staging CT scan shows retro-peritoneal lymphadenopathy but no nodes above the diaphragm.

2  A 30-year-old man with right-sided undescended testis develops a mass in the left testicle. Left orchidectomy shows seminoma. CT scan shows no evidence of spread.

3  A 35-year-old man develops a hard right testicular mass. He undergoes orchidectomy which shows it to be a seminoma. A Staging CT scan shows lymph node spread above and below the diaphragm.

## THEME: TYPES OF HERNIA

**A** Direct inguinal hernia

**B** Femoral hernia

**C** Indirect inguinal hernia

**D** Littre's hernia

**E** Lumbar hernia

**F** Paraumbilical hernia

**G** Spigelian hernia

**For each of the following scenarios, choose the most appropriate option from the list above. Each option may be used once, more than once or not at all.**

4  A 58-year-old man with previous laparotomy for diverticular disease develops a hernia at the lower end of his midline scar. The hernia becomes irreducible and he presents to A&E with severe pain. At operation the contents of the hernia show a strangulated Meckel's diverticulum.

5  A 52-year-old woman presents with a tender swelling in the left groin. Examination reveals that this is irreducible with a cough impulse, lying below and lateral to the pubic tubercle.

6  A 28-year-old man presents with a groin swelling, which is easily reducible and has a cough impulse. On standing the hernia descends into the scrotum. Reducing the hernia and placing pressure 1 cm above the mid-point of the inguinal ligament prevents the hernia from reappearing.

7  A 78-year-old man presents with a reducible mass just superior to the right iliac crest.

# THEME: BONE TUMOURS

**A** Angiosarcoma

**B** Chondrosarcoma

**C** Ewing's sarcoma

**D** Giant cell tumour

**E** Metastasis from lung carcinoma

**F** Myeloma

**G** Osteoblastoma

**H** Osteosarcoma

**For each of the following scenarios, choose the most likely diagnosis from the list above. Each option may be used once, more than once or not at all.**

8    A 15-year-old boy presents with a painful enlarging mass of the lower left femur. An X-ray shows a sclerotic lesion with periosteal elevation. The knee joint is not involved. Chest x-ray shows lesions suspicious of pulmonary metastases. He has a past medical history of retinoblastoma as a child.

9    A 60-year-old gentleman with a past history of multiple osteochondromas affecting the right proximal humerus and ribs presents with a slowly enlarging mass of the right humerus. The X-ray shows endosteal scalloping and cortical thickening. There is evidence of pulmonary spread on chest X-ray.

10    A 10-year-old girl presents with a tender enlarging mass affecting the diaphysis of the left femur. An X-ray shows this to be a lytic lesion. Biopsy identifies it as being a tumour of vascular endothelium.

11    An 80-year-old man with known Paget's disease affecting both legs presents with painful mass affecting the right tibia. An X-ray shows a lytic lesion arising from the medullary cavity. Pulmonary metastases are present on chest X-ray.

# THEME: MANAGEMENT OF ACUTE ISCHAEMIA

**A**　Amputation

**B**　Angioplasty

**C**　Embolectomy

**D**　Management of risk factors

**E**　Reconstruction

**F**　Thrombolysis

**G**　Watch and wait

**For each of the following scenarios, choose the most appropriate option from the list above. Each option may be used once, more than once or not at all.**

12　A 72-year-old man has history of atrial fibrillation but not of peripheral vascular disease or claudication pain. He presents to A&E with a 2-hour history of an acutely ischaemic left leg. Angiography shows a blockage at the origin of the left femoral artery.

13　An 84-year-old woman, who lives alone, presents with a 36-hour history of acute ischaemia of right foot. Angiography shows occlusion of the right superficial femoral artery.

14　A 64-year-old man, a heavy smoker, has a history of intermittent claudication affecting the right calf. He presents with an acutely ischaemic right leg. On examination the limb is found to be insensate. Angiogram shows occlusion of the right femoral artery with good distal run-off.

15　A 70-year-old woman has a history of acute on chronic ischaemic right leg. This was treated initially with thrombolysis which failed. An angiogram shows occlusion of the superficial femoral artery with poor distal run-off.

# THEME: JAUNDICE

**A** Hepatic jaundice
**B** Pre-hepatic jaundice
**C** Post-hepatic jaundice

**For each of the following scenarios, choose the most appropriate option from the list above. Each option may be used once, more than once or not at all.**

16    A 29-year-old man underwent open reduction and internal fixation of a femoral fracture following an RTA. His post-operative haemoglobin was 6.5 g/dl (65 g/l), so a blood transfusion was started. During administration of the first unit he develops pyrexia, rigors, dyspnoea, loin pain and jaundice.

17    A 60-year-old man who has just returned from a holiday in Thailand, presents with epigastric pain, nausea and vomiting, followed by the development of jaundice. Urine is dark and stools are pale.

18    A 25-year-old man, usually fit and well, develops jaundice on occasions, usually following a night out drinking. Investigations suggest Gilbert's syndrome.

19    A 36-year-old with schizophrenia develops jaundice 4 months after starting chlorpromazine.

# THEME: NECK LUMPS

**A** Branchial cyst
**B** Cystic hygroma
**C** Lymph node
**D** Lymphoma
**E** Thyroglossal cyst
**F** Thyroid carcinoma
**G** Toxic multi-nodular goitre

**For each of the following scenarios, choose the most appropriate diagnosis from the list above. Each option may be used once, more than once or not at all.**

20   A 12-year-old child presents with a painless midline neck swelling which is fluctuant on palpation. It moves both on swallowing and on protrusion of the tongue.

21   A 2-year-old boy presents with unilateral painless swelling at the base of the neck. It brilliantly transilluminates.

22   A 25-year-old woman presents with an irregular, painless midline neck swelling which moves on swallowing but not on protrusion of the tongue. She also complains of feeling anxious and sweaty, and has lost some weight in recent weeks.

23   A 35-year-old man presents with an enlarging neck lump between the junction of the upper and middle thirds of the anterior border of the left sternocleidomastoid muscle. The mass is non-tender.

24   A 69-year-old gentleman presents with weight loss, epigastric pain and a hard lump in the supraclavicular fossa.

# THEME: SURGICAL MANAGEMENT OF INFLAMMATORY BOWEL DISEASE

**A** Colectomy and ileo-rectal anastomosis

**B** Extended right hemicolectomy

**C** Ileo-caecal resection

**D** Proctocolectomy and ileo-anal pouch

**E** Proctocolectomy and ileostomy

**F** Stricturoplasty

**G** Subtotal colectomy + ileostomy + mucous fistula

For each of the following scenarios, choose the most appropriate option from the list above. Each option may be used once, more than once or not at all.

25 A 15-year-old boy with a history of ulcerative colitis for 5 years has a 2-year history of severe disease resulting in weight loss and growth failure. He is commenced on increasing doses of steroids without success. Disease is present from transverse colon to rectum.

26 A 39-year-old gentleman with ulcerative colitis presents with a severe acute exacerbation. Three days after admission he develops severe abdominal pain, becomes septic and on examination has a rigid abdomen with peritonism. Erect chest X-ray shows air under the diaphragm.

27 A 27-year-old woman with Crohn's disease is admitted for the fourth occasion in 6 months with small bowel obstruction. Barium follow through shows a 4 cm stricture of proximal ileum.

28 A 22-year-old woman with diagnosis of Crohn's disease has a history over the past year of recurrent anaemia and weight loss. Colonoscopy shows severe inflammation and active disease affecting the caecum and terminal ileum. Maximum medical therapy has been unsuccessful.

29    A 21-year-old patient with a history of severe ulcerative colitis has failed on medical treatment alone. Investigations show rectal sparing.

# THEME: SCROTAL SWELLINGS

**A**  Acute epididymo-orchitis

**B**  Encysted hydrocoele of cord

**C**  Epididymal cyst

**D**  Chronic epididymo-orchitis

**E**  Haematocele

**F**  Hydrocoele

**G**  Inguino-scrotal hernia

**H**  Sebaceous cyst

**I**  Testicular tumour

**J**  Varicocele

**For each of the following scenarios, choose the most appropriate option from the list above. Each option may be used once, more than once or not at all.**

30    A 42-year-old man presents with a non-tender right scrotal swelling which has been gradually increasing in size over several months. On examination it is fluctuant and transilluminates. It is not possible to feel the right testicle separately from the swelling, but it is possible to get above it and feel the cord as a separate structure.

31    A 65-year-old man presents with a slowly enlarging painless scrotal swelling. On examination it is fluctuant and transilluminates. It is possible to get above it on examination and feel the testis as a separate structure. The swelling is found to lie above and slightly behind the testis.

32    A 70-year-old man has a history of a long-standing 'aching' sensation in the right testis. On examination he has a firm craggy mass and a few discharging sinuses on the scrotal skin. Urine microscopy shows sterile pyuria.

33    A 38-year-old man presents with a left-sided scrotal swelling. On examination it is a soft, compressible swelling which does not have a cough impulse. It is not possible to get above it and it disappears on lying down.

34    A 45-year-old man presents with a right-sided scrotal swelling which increases in size on standing up. On examination it is not transilluminable and it is not possible to get above it. There is a positive cough impulse.

35    A 25-year-old man presents with a smooth left-sided painless scrotal swelling which is transilluminable and fluctuant. It is possible to feel the testis as a separate structure below the swelling.

## THEME: UPPER LIMB FRACTURES

**A** Barton's fracture

**B** Bennett's fracture

**C** Colles' fracture

**D** Galeazzi's fracture

**E** Monteggia's fracture

**F** Smith's fracture

**For each of the following scenarios, choose the most appropriate option from the list above. Each option may be used once, more than once or not at all.**

36  A 24-year-old woman presents with a painful left arm following an RTA. The X-ray shows a fracture of the upper third of the ulna together with an associated dislocated radial head.

37  An 84-year-old woman has a fall in the street landing on her right hand which appears swollen and deformed. An X-ray shows a fracture of the distal radius which is angulated dorsally. The fracture extends intra-articularly and there is subluxation of the carpus.

38  A 76-year-old woman stumbles down the stairs at home landing heavily on her left arm. On examination she has a deformed, bruised left wrist. An X-ray shows an extra-articular fracture of the distal radius which is displaced volarly.

39  A 15-year-old boy is knocked off his bicycle and lands on his right arm. He presents to A&E with a swollen tender wrist. An X-ray shows a facture of the mid-shaft of the radius and dislocation of the inferior radio-ulnar joint.

## THEME: STAGING OF COLON CANCER

A   Duke's A stage

B   Duke's B stage

C   Duke's C stage

D   Duke's D stage

E   None of the above

**For each of the following clinical scenarios, select the most appropriate answer. Each answer may be used once, more than once or not at all.**

40   A 68-year-old man presents with weight loss and iron deficiency anaemia. Colonoscopy confirms a caecal mass. The specimen obtained at laparotomy shows adenocarcinoma extending through the bowel wall. All of the nine lymph nodes removed are involved.

41   A 52-year-old man presents with a history of increasingly severe constipation and rectal bleeding. He is found to have a stenosing lesion of the distal sigmoid colon. Biopsy confirms adenocarcinoma. He undergoes anterior resection and the specimen shows three out of the total seven nodes removed are involved.

42   A 25-year-old man from a family known to carry the *HNPCC* gene is found to have a lesion in the transverse colon at colonoscopy. Resection and histological examination of the specimen shows this to be invading the muscle layer of the bowel wall.

# THEME: URINARY SYSTEM TRAUMA

**A** Catheterisation and contrast
**B** CT scan
**C** Cystogram
**D** Retrograde uteropyelography
**E** Surgical exploration
**F** Urethrogram

**For each of the following scenarios, choose the most appropriate investigation from the list above. Each option may be used once, more than once or not at all.**

43 A 25-year-old man slips while walking along the top of a metal gate and falls straddling the gate. On examination he is in significant pain and has butterfly pattern bruising to the perineum. There is fresh blood at the urethral meatus.

44 A 30-year-old man involved in a fight sustains a blow to the groin with a blunt instrument. On examination there is gross swelling and bruising with an area of tense swelling around the left testicle which is becoming increasingly large and painful.

45 A 52-year-old man is mugged and stabbed with a knife in the area of the left renal angle. He complains of loin pain. Dipstick shows microscopic haematuria.

# THEME: PREPARATION OF PATIENTS FOR ENDOCRINE SURGERY

**A** Bowel preparation

**B** Calcitonin infusion

**C** Corticosteroids

**D** Phenoxybenzamine and propranolol

**E** Thallium technetium scan

**F** Thyroxine

**G** Vocal cord examination

**For each of the following scenarios, choose the most appropriate option from the list above. Each option may be used once, more than once or not at all.**

46 A 28-year-old woman with Graves' disease resistant to medical treatment is due to have a subtotal thyroidectomy for symptoms of compression.

47 A 42-year-old patient is planned to have a parathyroidectomy after presenting with raised calcium and parathyroid hormone levels with no history of renal disease.

48 A 34-year-old patient is found to have bilateral adrenal masses on CT, and suspected to have phaeochromocytoma. An adrenalectomy is planned.

# THEME: MANAGEMENT OF PAEDIATRIC DISORDERS

**A** Broad-spectrum antibiotics

**B** Gastrografin enema

**C** Laparotomy and duodenostomy

**D** Laparotomy and proceed

**E** Pneumatic reduction

**F** Ramstedt's pyloromyotomy

For each of the following scenarios, choose the most appropriate management option from the list above. Each option may be used once, more than once or not at all.

49 A 40-day-old baby develops projectile vomiting approximately 20 minutes after each feed together with failure to thrive. On examination an olive-shaped mass is noted in the RUQ following feeding. Bloods show a metabolic alkalosis.

50 A 2-day-old baby known to have cystic fibrosis presents with a distended abdomen and bilious vomiting. His rectum is empty.

51 A 1-year-old infant presents with intermittent spasms of abdominal pain associated with drawing up of the legs and a small amount of rectal bleeding. A sausage-shaped mass is noted in the epigastrium. Two similar episodes in the past were treated with hydrostatic reduction.

# THEME: RENAL STONES

A   Extracorporal shock wave lithotripsy (ESWL)

B   Nephrectomy

C   Percutaneous nephrolithotomy (PCNL)

D   Rigid ureteroscopy

E   Watch and wait

For each of the following scenarios, choose the most appropriate management option from the list above. Each option may be used once, more than once or not at all.

52   A 54-year-old woman with a history of renal stone disease presents with a 2-month history of intermittent left loin pain. An intravenous urogram (IVU) shows a 1.5 cm stone in the left renal pelvis but no evidence of obstruction. She has a past history of ischaemic heart disease and has a 4 cm aortic aneurysm lying close to the origin of the left renal artery; this is under surveillance.

53   A 27-year-old man presents to A&E with severe right loin and groin pain and microscopic haematuria on dipstick. Pain is well controlled with NSAIDs and pethidine. An IVU confirms the presence of a 4 mm stone in the right mid-ureter region.

54   A 42-year-old man presents to A&E with severe right loin pain radiating to the groin. He is sweating profusely and vomiting with a temperature of 38.9 °C. Dipstick shows 3+ blood and 3+ leucocytes. An IVU shows a 5 mm stone in the upper right ureter and dilated calyces.

55   A 24-year-old woman develops severe loin pain with one episode of frank haematuria. She is apyrexial. An IVU shows a 1 cm calculus lying in the lower pole of the right kidney.

# THEME: MANAGEMENT OF THYROID CANCER

**A** Chemotherapy alone

**B** Lobectomy

**C** Subtotal thyroidectomy

**D** Surgery and external beam radiotherapy

**E** Total thyroidectomy and thyroxine replacement

**For each of the following scenarios, choose the most appropriate treatment option from the list above. Each option may be used once, more than once or not at all.**

56  A 27-year-old man with history of previous neck irradiation for lymphoma presents with thyroid mass. Fine needle aspiration reveals cells with 'Orphan Annie' nuclei. CT shows localised disease.

57  A 90-year-old woman presents with hard thyroid mass and a progressively hoarse voice. Cervical lymph nodes are hard and enlarged.

58  A 48-year-old patient with a family history of multiple endocrine dysplasia (MEN) syndrome presents with a thyroid mass that appears malignant but shows no evidence of spread.

59  A 57-year-old woman presents with painless thyroid swelling and weight loss. Fine needle aspiration of the swelling indicates that it is a lymphoma.

## THEME: PRURITUS ANI

**A**   Anal carcinoma

**B**   Anal fissure

**C**   Anal polyp

**D**   Fistula-in-ano

**E**   Gonorrhoea

**F**   Haemorrhoids

**G**   Syphilis

**H**   Yeast infection

**For each of the following scenarios, choose the most appropriate option from the list above. Each option may be used once, more than once or not at all.**

60   A 35-year-old woman who regularly takes codeine-based analgesics for tension headaches presents with pruritus ani, rectal bleeding and severe pain following defaecation.

61   A 57-year-old HIV-positive man has a history of long-standing AIN but was lost to follow-up for the past 5 years. He now presents with pruritus ani and a firm ulcerated mass at the anal margin with palpable lymph nodes.

62   A 25-year-old woman with a history of ulcerative colitis on maximum medical therapy to help control disease presents with pruritus ani. On examination the peri-anal area is red, inflamed and excoriated with a well-demarcated edge.

63   A 48-year-old man presents with a 3-month history of weight loss and intermittent fever. He also complains of itching around the anus, associated with soreness and purulent discharge.

# THEME: MANAGEMENT OF VENOUS DISEASE OF THE LOWER LIMB

**A** Debridement and compression bandaging

**B** Elevation and NSAIDs

**C** Injection sclerotherapy

**D** Sapheno-femoral ligation

**E** Split-skin graft

**F** Stab avulsions

**G** Systemic antibiotics

**H** Topical antibiotics

For each of the following scenarios, choose the most appropriate option from the list above. Each option may be used once, more than once or not at all.

64  A 46-year-old woman has long-standing varicose veins affecting both legs which have recently started to ache. Doppler examination shows no problem with the deep venous system. Varicosities are in the distribution of the long saphenous vein.

65  A 69-year-old woman has a history of deep vein thrombosis affecting the right leg 20 years ago. She now presents with long-standing ulcers over the right gaiter region. ABPI of both legs = 0.8. She is treated with debridement and compression dressing, but review at 12 weeks shows no improvement.

66  An 84-year-old woman with a long-standing venous ulcer of the left shin, treated with regular debridement and dressings, notices it is becoming increasingly tender. On examination the ulcer has a small amount of purulent, offensive discharge and there is surrounding cellulitis.

67  A 60-year-old woman with a 10-year history of varicose veins affecting both legs presents with an acute episode of painful thrombophlebitis.

# THEME: PAEDIATRIC ORTHOPAEDIC DISORDERS

**A** Congenital dysplasia of the hip
**B** Congenital talipes equinovarus
**C** Irritable hip
**D** Perthes' disease
**E** Septic arthritis
**F** Slipped upper femoral epiphysis (SUFE)
**G** Tuberculosis

For each of the following scenarios, choose the most likely diagnosis from the list above. Each option may be used once, more than once or not at all.

68    A 4-year-old boy presents with vague pain in left hip and thigh. Examination reveals a reduced level of internal rotation and abduction. X-ray shows flattening and deformity of the femoral head.

69    A 15-year-old overweight boy complains of right knee pain which has recently got much worse. The right leg is shortened and externally rotated. Anteroposterior (AP) views of knee and hip joints are normal.

70    A 3-year-old girl presents with a sudden-onset limp affecting the right leg. She appears well, not complaining of any pain and is apyrexial. Bloods and X-rays are all normal.

# THEME: ABDOMINAL SIGNS

**A** Battles' sign

**B** Boas' sign

**C** Cullen's sign

**D** Grey Turner's sign

**E** Murphy's sign

**F** Psoas stretch sign

**G** Rovsing's sign

**For each of the following clinical scenarios, choose the most appropriate option from the list above. Each answer may be used once, more than once or not at all.**

71    A 39-year-old man presents to A&E with severe epigastric and right upper quadrant (RUQ) pain radiating through to the back, and associated with nausea and vomiting. Inspection of the abdomen shows bruising around the umbilicus.

72    A 54-year-old alcoholic is found collapsed at home in a state of shock. She is unable to give a history but shouts out when her abdomen is palpated. Amylase is 3000 somogyi u/dL, erect chest X-ray normal. A bluish discoloration is noticed around the flanks.

73    A 45-year-old woman with known gallstones presents with RUQ pain, fever and is found to have a raised white count. On palpation of the abdomen she is found to be tender in the RUQ and this increases when she breathes in such that it causes her to stop inspiring.

## THEME: ABDOMINAL INCISIONS

**A** Gridiron incision

**B** Kocher's incision

**C** Lanz incision

**D** Laparoscopic port incisions

**E** Midline incision

**F** Paramedian incision

**G** Pfannenstiel's incision

**H** Rooftop incision

**I** Rutherford-Morrison incision

**For each of the following clinical scenarios, choose the most appropriate incision. Each option may be used once, more than once or not at all.**

74   A 36-year-old woman presents with abdominal distension. A CT scan reveals a benign-looking right ovarian cyst, 5 × 5 cm. An elective excision is planned.

75   A 38-year-old alcoholic presents with severe epigastric pain. Examination reveals a rigid abdomen and no bowel sounds. Erect chest X-ray shows air under the diaphragm.

76   A 38-year-old woman who is 10 weeks pregnant has had multiple episodes of cholecystitis in recent months which are becoming increasingly frequent. She is to have cholecystectomy as soon as possible.

77   A 16-year-old girl presents with central abdominal pain which shifts to the right iliac fossa and is associated with nausea and diarrhoea. She has a low grade temperature and white cell count of $18 \times 10^9$. Examination reveals rebound tenderness and guarding in the right iliac fossa.

78   A 48-year-old woman admitted for curative surgery for carcinoma of the head of the pancreas.

# THEME: FULL BLOOD COUNT

Normal values: Haemoglobin (Hb) 11.5–16.5 g/dl (women), 13–18g/dl (men); mean corpuscular volume (MCV) 78–98 fL; white blood cell (WBC) count 4–11 $\times 10^9$/l; neutrophils 2.0–7.5 $\times 10^9$/l; eosinophils 0.05–0.35 $\times 10^9$/l; platelets 150–400 $\times 10^9$/l

Table 1

|   | Hb | MCV | WBC count | Neutrophils | Eosinophils | Platelets |
|---|-----|-----|-----------|-------------|-------------|-----------|
| A | 10.0 | 120 | 9.0 | 6.0 | 0.1 | 300 |
| B | 7.0 | 80 | 8.0 | 5.0 | 0.2 | 250 |
| C | 6.0 | 60 | 7.0 | 4.0 | 0.1 | 170 |
| D | 13.5 | 90 | 19.0 | 16.0 | 0.1 | 290 |
| E | 22 | 87 | 5.0 | 2.5 | 0.3 | 350 |
| F | 15.0 | 89 | 14.0 | 7.5 | 4.0 | 350 |

For each of the following scenarios, choose the most appropriate full blood count (FBC) result from the table above. Each option may be used once, more than once or not at all.

79  An 18-year-old girl returns from gap year in Africa with fever, abdominal pain and diarrhoea. Positive stool sample indicates amoebic dysentery.

80  A 67-year-old chronic alcoholic.

81  A 55-year-old woman on intravenous steroid therapy.

82  A 66-year-old man diagnosed with friable tumour in the right colon on colonoscopy.

83  A 33-year-old man, known to have hereditary elliptocytosis (haemolytic anaemia).

84  A 75-year-old hypertensive man with diagnosis of polycythemia rubra vera.

## THEME: GALLSTONE DISEASE

**A**   Conservative management

**B**   Endoscopic retrograde cholangiopancreatography (ERCP) and sphincterotomy

**C**   Laparoscopic cholecystectomy

**D**   Open cholecystectomy

**E**   T-tube insertion

**For each of the following scenarios, choose the most appropriate management option from the list above. Each option may be used once, more than once or not at all.**

85   A 36-year-old woman presents to A&E with RUQ pain becoming increasingly severe after a fatty meal. She has a fever and a raised white cell count but her amylase is normal. Ultrasound scan confirms multiple gallstones in the gallbladder.

86   A 45-year-old obese, diabetic woman with a previous history of laparotomy for perforated duodenal ulcer is seen in outpatient clinic 2 months following her sixth hospital admission for acute cholecystitis in the past 5 years.

87   A 67-year-old man with known gallstones presents to hospital with severe epigastric and RUQ pain associated with nausea and vomiting. He is apyrexial and white cell count and amylase are normal. The pain settles with a strong analgesic.

# THEME: SALIVARY GLANDS

**A** Parotid gland

**B** Sublingual gland

**C** Submandibular gland

**For each of the following scenarios, choose the most appropriate option from the list above. Each answer may be used once, more than once or not at all.**

88 The facial nerve runs through this gland and its blood supply comes from a branch of the external carotid artery. Of tumours arising in this gland, 80% are benign.

89 This gland secretes mucous and serous saliva. Secretomotor fibres come from the parasympathetic system which hitchhike along with the chorda tympani and lingual nerve.

90 This gland is divided into deep and superficial parts by the posterior border of the mylohyoid muscle. Blood supply comes from the facial artery and vein.

# THEME: MANAGEMENT OF HERNIAS

**A** Conservative management

**B** Elective hernia repair

**C** Emergency hernia repair

**D** Urgent hernia repairs, ie on an elective list but prioritised over benign conditions

**For each of the following scenarios, choose the most appropriate course of action from the list above. Each option may be used once, more than once or not at all.**

91 A 79-year-old woman presents to clinic with a small non-tender lump in her groin. It has been present for the past 2 months. It is non-tender and measures approximately 3 cm in diameter. It lies below and lateral to the pubic tubercle. It is irreducible and there is no cough impulse.

92 A 1-year-old boy presents with a small indirect inguinal hernia.

93 A 65-year-old man presents with an indirect inguinal hernia. It is non-tender and has been present for 3 weeks. It initially reduced spontaneously, but over the past 2 days it has not been reducible.

94 An 84-year-old man with chronic bronchitis, diabetes mellitus and a past medical history of two episodes of myocardial infarction presents with an inguinal hernia. It has been present for 7 years, but since the past day it has been very painful and irreducible. On examination it is tender, erythematous and there is no cough impulse.

95 A healthy 84-year-old man presents to clinic with a small right inguinal hernia. On examination there is a 2 cm diameter direct hernia which is palpable only on coughing.

# THEME: STATISTICS

A  4%

B  5%

C  10%

D  20%

E  24%

F  25%

G  75%

H  76%

I  80%

J  90%

K  95%

L  96%

A new test is developed for detecting *Chlamydia*. In a trial 200 people are tested. The test produces 100 positive results and 100 negative results. Of the 100 positive results, 4 are false positives. Of the 100 negative results, 24 are false negatives. From the list above, choose the option to the nearest per cent. You may use each option once, more than once or not at all.

What is the:

( )  96  Specificity

( )  97  Sensitivity

( )  98  Negative predictive value (NPV)

( )  99  Positive predictive value (PPV)

## THEME: PANCREATIC TUMOURS

A  Gastrinoma

B  Glucagonoma

C  Insulinoma

D  Somatostatinoma

E  VIPoma

For each of the following scenarios, choose the most appropriate likely tumour from the list above. Each option may be used once, more than once or not at all.

100  A 43-year-old man with known parathyroid adenoma presents to casualty with haematemesis.

101  A 64-year-old woman presents with obstructive jaundice and RUQ pain. A random blood glucose is 15.4 mmol/l and an ultrasound scan of the abdomen reveals gallstones.

102  A 42-year-old woman presents with weight loss and anaemia. A random blood glucose is 15.2 mmol/l.

# THEME: BREAST INVESTIGATIONS

**A** Core biopsy

**B** CT scan

**C** Fine needle aspiration

**D** Magnetic resonance imaging (MRI)

**E** No further investigation

**F** Ultrasound-guided fine needle aspiration

**G** Ultrasound scan

**For each of the following scenarios, choose the most appropriate investigation from the list above. Each option may be used once, more than once or not at all.**

103 A 40-year-old woman presents with a painless, enlarging lump in her neck and dysphagia. The lump is easily palpable, moves up with swallowing and measures approximately 6 cm in diameter.

104 A 28-year-old woman presents with a right-sided breast lump. It measures 1 cm in diameter, is mobile, smooth, non-tender, and is superficial to the pectoralis major. There are no associated skin changes. Both axillae are clear. An ultrasound scan is reported as showing a benign lump.

105 A 55-year-old woman is sent to your clinic after screening mammography reveals a suspicious area in the left breast. Clinical examination does not reveal any suspicious areas.

# THEME: INTRAVENOUS FLUIDS

**A**  0.45% Sodium chloride solution

**B**  0.9% Sodium chloride solution

**C**  4% Dextrose/0.18% sodium chloride solution

**D**  5% Dextrose solution

**E**  Compound sodium lactate solution

**F**  Dextran 70

**For each of the following questions, choose the most appropriate fluid from the list above. Each option may be used once, more than once or not at all.**

106  Which fluid has been shown to reduce the incidence of deep venous thrombosis?

107  Which fluid is recommended in the Advanced Trauma Life Support (ATLS) guidelines for the initial resuscitation of the trauma patient?

108  Which fluid contains 5 mmol of potassium per litre?

109  Which fluid contains 150 mmol of sodium per litre?

110  Which fluid given in equal volumes expands the intravascular compartment least?

# THEME: SPECIFIC TESTS

**A**   Allen's test

**B**   Froment's test

**C**   Lachman's test

**D**   Pivot shift

**E**   Simmonds' test

**F**   Tinel's test

**G**   Trendelenburg's test

**Which test would give the most appropriate information in the following scenarios? Each option may be used once, more than once or not at all.**

111   A 21-year-old, very anxious footballer presents to fracture clinic with an acute swelling of the right knee following a twisting injury 2 days ago. There is no bony tenderness around the knee joint. He is able to fully weight bear, fully extend his knee and flex to 90 degrees. Aspiration confirms a haemarthrosis.

112   A 69-year-old woman attends outpatients. On examination she has guttering in the dorsal aspect of her right hand and apparent wasting of the muscles of the hand.

113   A 35-year-old man attends A&E with acute, severe pain in the right calf. He finds it difficult to walk, and cannot plantar flex his right foot.

# THEME: CALCULI

**A** Bile pigment stone

**B** Calcium oxalate

**C** Calcium phosphate

**D** Cholesterol stone

**E** Cystine stone

**F** Urate

**For each of the following scenarios, choose the most likely substance for stone formation from the list above. Each option may be used once, more than once or not at all.**

114 A 32-year-old man presents with haematuria. A KUB (kidney-ureter-bladder) X-ray reveals a staghorn calculus in the right kidney and a mid-stream urine sample grows proteus.

115 A 31-year-old woman with known sickle cell anaemia attends A&E with biliary colic. X-rays show the presence of stones in the gallbladder.

116 A 28-year-old man presents with ureteric colic. A KUB shows a stone at the right vesico-ureteric junction.

# THEME: NECK LUMPS

**A** Branchial cyst

**B** Cervical rib

**C** Chemodectoma

**D** Cystic hygroma

**E** Lymph nodes

**F** Multi-nodular goitre

**G** Pharyngeal pouch

**H** Thyroglossal cyst

**For each of the following scenarios, choose the most appropriate diagnosis from the list above. Each option may be used once, more than once or not at all.**

117 A 25-year-old woman presents with a painless lump in her neck. It lies in the midline 2 cm above the thyroid cartilage, moves up on swallowing and on protrusion of the tongue.

118 A 50-year-old man attends complaining of a painless lump in the neck. On examination a 4 cm smooth firm lump is found to be in the upper part of the anterior triangle of the neck. It is pulsatile and on further questioning the patient admits to a number of recent black-outs.

119 A 20-year-old attends with a large cystic lesion in the posterior triangle of the neck. It is fluctuant and on examination with a torch, translucent.

120 A 23-year-old attends complaining of multiple neck lumps. She also has a sore throat, fever and splenomegaly.

# THEME: TYPES OF ULCER

**A**  Arterial ulcer

**B**  Curling's ulcer

**C**  Cushing's ulcer

**D**  Duodenal ulcer

**E**  Gastric ulcer

**F**  Marjolin's ulcer

**G**  Rodent ulcer

**H**  Venous ulcer

**For each of the following scenarios, choose the most appropriate option from the list above. Each option may be used once, more than once or not at all.**

121  A 43-year-old man is admitted to the ICU following an RTA. He has been unconscious and intubated since having a subdural haematoma evacuated. On day 4 of his admission he begins to have blood aspirated from his nasogastric tube.

122  A 76-year-old woman presents to clinic with a large ulcer over her medial malleolus. She has recently noticed that it has grown and bleeds more easily. On examination it has a friable centre and raised edges.

123  An 84-year-old man presents with a small ulcer on the bridge of his nose. It has been present for a number of months. On examination it has pearly white, rolled edges.

124  A 24-year-old has 24% third-degree burns. Three days after his admission he complains of melaena.

# THEME: SKIN LESIONS

**A**  Basal cell carcinoma

**B**  Dermatofibroma

**C**  Keratoacanthoma

**D**  Melanoma

**E**  Pyoderma gangrenosum

**F**  Pyogenic granuloma

**G**  Squamous cell carcinoma

**H**  Strawberry naevus

**For each of the following scenarios, choose the most likely diagnosis from the list above. Each option may be used once, more than once or not at all.**

125  A 40-year-old woman presents with a lump on the anterior aspect of the leg. It has been slowly growing over the past 3 years and is now causing cosmetic disfigurement. On examination you find a 1 cm smooth, firm disc.

126  A 2-year-old child is brought to clinic with a small 1 cm lump in her hairline. The lump has been present since birth, but recently it has begun to bleed. On examination the lump is sessile, dark red and has a small ulcerated area in its centre.

127  A 76-year-old woman presents with a lesion on her left cheek. There is a small ulcer with a raised pearly edge. She reports that it has been scabbing over, with the scab falling off every now and then.

128  A 31-year-old man presents with a mole on his right shoulder. It has grown over the past 2 months and is very itchy. It bleeds occasionally. On examination there is a 2 cm irregular mole on the shoulder with a surrounding brown halo. He is also jaundiced.

129   A 28-year-old man presents with a lump on the dorsum of his left hand. The lump has grown rapidly over the past 2 weeks. It bleeds easily and is discharging serous fluid. He gives a history of minor trauma to the same hand 3 weeks before. The lump is not painful. On examination there is a bright red, soft, 1 cm hemispherical lump present.

130   A 64-year-old woman presents with a non-painful lump on her left arm. It has grown rapidly over the past 2 weeks. On examination it is approximately 2 cm in diameter and has a central brown core. It is firm in consistency, but the central core is hard.

# THEME: AIRWAY MANAGEMENT

**A** Bag-valve-mask

**B** Double-lumen cuffed endotracheal tube

**C** Nasopharyngeal airway

**D** Needle cricothyroidotomy

**E** Oropharyngeal airway

**F** Percutaneous tracheostomy

**G** Single-lumen cuffed endotracheal tube

**H** Single-lumen uncuffed endotracheal tube

**For each of the situations below, choose the most appropriate airway adjunct from the list above. Each option may be used once, more than once or not at all.**

131  A 7-year-old child is brought in to A&E having been rescued from a house fire. He is in respiratory distress and there is evidence of soot around his nasal passages.

132  A 64-year-old man due to undergo elective repair of a thoracic aortic aneurysm.

133  You are the only doctor in the A&E department. A patient with severe facial injuries suffered in an RTA is brought in by paramedics. He goes into respiratory arrest and an initial attempt at endotracheal intubation fails.

134  A 76-year-old man is on the ICU following emergency laparotomy. He is expected to remain on the ICU for another week.

135  A 27-year-old man involved in a house fire is brought to A&E. He has some singeing of his nasal hair. His respiratory rate is 28 breaths/min, and pulse oximetry gives a reading of 94% on 4 l/min oxygen.

# THEME: COLORECTAL CARCINOMA PROCEDURES

**A** Abdomino-perineal resection

**B** Anterior resection

**C** DeLorme's procedure

**D** Extended right hemicolectomy

**E** Hartmann's procedure

**F** Right hemicolectomy

**For each of the following situations, choose the most appropriate operation from the list above. Each option may be used once, more than once or not at all.**

136 A patient with carcinoma of the sigmoid colon presenting with peritonitis due to a perforation.

137 A 68-year-old man presents with rectal bleeding. Colonoscopy reveals a caecal tumour.

138 A 76-year-old woman presents with rectal bleeding. Digital rectal examination reveals a tumour 2 cm from the anal margin. This is confirmed by proctoscopy.

139 A 54-year-old woman presents with acute appendicitis. A tumour is found in the appendix at appendicoectomy.

140 A 64-year-old man presents with small bowel obstruction. He gives a 2-month history of a weight loss of 12 kg (2 stone) and intermittent rectal bleeding.

141 An 88-year-old man is found to have a 2 cm tumour of the sigmoid colon. His past medical history includes diabetes mellitus, two episodes of myocardial infarction and peripheral vascular disease.

# THEME: PROSTATISM

**A** Alfuzosin

**B** Antibiotics

**C** Radical prostatectomy

**D** Subcapsular orchidectomy

**E** Tolterodine

**F** TURP

**G** Zolendronic acid

For each of the following scenarios, choose the most appropriate treatment option from the list above. Each option may be used once, more than once or not at all.

142 A 72-year-old man complains of acute abdominal pain 1 day post total knee replacement. A urinary catheter is passed with difficulty and initially drains 850 ml of urine. His pain is relieved. His PSA is 36 nmol/ml.

143 An 84-year-old man with known carcinoma of the prostate returns to clinic complaining of severe back pain. A bone scan shows multiple vertebral metastases, though none causing spinal cord compression. He has previously been treated with subcapsular orchidectomy and bicalutamide. His PSA is 432 nmol/ml.

144 A 64-year-old man returns to clinic and continues to complain of poor flow, incomplete emptying, nocturia and frequency of micturition despite treatment with tamsulosin and finasteride. His PSA is 4.2 nmol/ml. His post-void bladder scan reveals a residual urine of 568 ml.

145 A 64-year-old man complains of increased frequency of micturition, urgency and nocturia. He passes urine hourly. Uroflowmetry reveals a maximum flow rate of 26 ml/s.

## THEME: THE LIMPING CHILD

**A**  Developmental dysplasia of the hip (DDH)

**B**  Irritable hip

**C**  Osteomyelitis

**D**  Perthes' disease

**E**  Septic arthritis

**F**  SUFE

**For each of the following scenarios, choose the most likely diagnosis from the list above. Each option may be used once, more than once or not at all.**

146  A 4-year-old boy presents with a sudden-onset limp. There is no history of trauma. On arrival to A&E, he is flushed, dehydrated and pyrexial. All movements of his right hip appear to cause pain. Routine blood tests reveal a white cell count of $15.1 \times 10^9$, CRP 234 mg/L and ESR 65 mm/h.

147  A 16-year-old boy presents with a limp to the right-hand side. There is no history of trauma. He complains of pain around his right knee, and painful movements of the right knee and hip. He appears small for his age, and has no pubertal hair. On examination he has a full although painful range of movement in his right knee. Movements of the right hip are painful and internal rotation is restricted by 20 degrees.

148  An 18-month-old girl with a limp is referred by her general practitioner. She has just started walking. She is otherwise fit and well, and is up to date with all her vaccinations. Peri-natal history includes breech delivery and the parents report a club foot which was treated by physiotherapists when she was a neonate.

# THEME: STERILISATION

**A**  Glutaraldehyde 2%

**B**  Hot air sterilisation 160 °C for 2 hours

**C**  Irradiation

**D**  Steam sterilisation – 15 minutes at 121 °C

**E**  Steam sterilisation – 15 minutes at 134 °C

**For each of the following situations, choose the most appropriate form of sterilisation from the list above. You may use each option once, more than once or not at all.**

149  Sterilisation of a minor instrument set.

150  Sterilisation of a colonoscope.

151  Sterilisation of single-use stapling gun.

# THEME: TYPES OF SHOCK

A  Anaphylactic shock
B  Cardiogenic shock
C  Class I haemorrhagic shock
D  Class II haemorrhagic shock
E  Class III haemorrhagic shock
F  Class IV haemorrhagic shock
G  Neurogenic shock
H  Spinal shock

For each of the following scenarios, choose the most the most likely diagnosis from the list above. Each option may be used once, more than once or not at all.

152  A 21-year-old is brought to A&E. He was thrown off his motorbike at high speed. He was wearing a helmet. He has obvious bilateral open femoral fractures. He has a heart rate of 134 beats/min and a blood pressure of 76/52 mmHg. His respiratory rate is 36 breaths/min and he is extremely agitated.

153  A 39-year-old is involved in an RTA. He was the front seat passenger and was wearing a seat belt. He is complaining of severe chest pain. On examination he has a visible seatbelt mark across the front of his chest. He is tachycardic, with a heart rate of 124 beats/min, has a respiratory rate of 24 breaths/min and a blood pressure of 88/58 mmHg. His central venous pressure is 17 mmHg.

154 A 47-year-old is brought in following a motorbike accident. On admission he is conscious, lucid and has an open tibial fracture. His heart rate is 120 beats/min and his blood pressure is 139/85 mmHg. Over the next hour his blood pressure remains stable and his heart rate drops to 92 beats/min. He is given tetanus cover and antibiotics, and his wounds are dressed in povidone iodine (Betadine)-soaked gauze. He suddenly loses consciousness and his blood pressure drops to 70/40 mmHg. His heart rate increases to 128 beats/min.

155 An agitated 35-year-old woman is brought to A&E. She has been involved in an RTA. Her heart rate is 114 beats/min, respiratory rate 26 breaths/min and her blood pressure is 126/100 mmHg.

# THEME: PAEDIATRIC ABDOMINAL DISORDERS

**A**   Acute appendicitis

**B**   Constipation

**C**   Crohn's disease

**D**   Hirschsprung's disease

**E**   Intussusception

**F**   Mesenteric adenitis

**G**   Pyloric stenosis

**For each of the following scenarios, choose the most likely diagnosis from the list above. Each option may be used once, more than once or not at all.**

156   A 2-year-old boy with Down's syndrome presents with abdominal pain. On questioning his parents you find out that he has not passed stool for 10 days. He normally passes stools twice a week and seems to have frequent episodes of abdominal pain.

157   A 9-month-old baby presents with an acute abdomen. Parents report passage of a jelly-like red stool, and on examination there is a sausage-like mass in the upper abdomen.

158   A 15-year-old boy presents with a 6-week history of RIF pain which suddenly worsened in the past two days. He also reports the occasional passage of blood in this period.

## THEME: CONSENT

**A**  Accept wishes for non-treatment

**B**  Obtain consent from next of kin

**C**  Proceed to treat without consent of patient

**D**  Section under mental health act to treat

**E**  Seek second opinion

**F**  Requires order from court of law to treat

**For each of the following situations, choose the most appropriate option from the list above. Each option may be used once, more than once or not at all.**

159  A 43-year-old man with chronic depression attends with sudden onset abdominal pain. He is peritonitic and has air under his diaphragm. Your consultant has asked you to obtain consent for a laparotomy. The patient refuses and states he would rather die.

160  A 13-year-old has an off-ended distal radial and ulna fracture. On examination she has signs of median nerve compromise. You have spoken with both the girl and her mother and informed them that an operation is necessary. The mother is happy to proceed. The child is adamant that she does not wish to have an operation even though she might not regain full use of her hand.

161  An 84-year-old with known multi–infarct dementia has a fractured neck of femur. He keeps shouting that he wants to be left alone to die.

162  A 64-year-old man is brought into A&E unconscious. He is thought to have a perforated peptic ulcer secondary to non-steroidal anti–inflammatory drug (NSAID) use. He is known to have metastatic carcinoma of the prostate. His wife attends with an advance directive stating that he does not wish any form of surgery or resuscitation.

# THEME: UROLOGICAL INVESTIGATIONS

**A** Abdominal ultrasound

**B** CT Scan

**C** Intravenous urography

**D** Plain radiograph (KUB)

**E** Radionucleotide imaging

**F** Transrectal ultrasound

**G** Uroflowmetry

**H** Video urodynamics

For each of the following scenarios, choose the most appropriate investigation from the list above. Each option may be used once, more than once or not at all.

163  A 64-year-old man is referred by his general practitioner with a PSA of 11.0 ng/mL. DRE reveals a 50 g craggy-feeling prostate.

164  A 84-year-old man with known metastatic carcinoma of the prostate attends A&E. He is complaining of abdominal pain and has not passed urine in 18 hours. Clinical examination reveals a tender abdomen, with increased tenderness around the renal angles. DRE reveals a 50 g craggy prostate. He is catheterised and has a residual volume of 35 ml.

165  A 46-year-old man presents with a single episode of haematuria. Flexible cystoscopy is performed in clinic revealing normal looking bladder and urethral mucosa.

166  A 17-year-old boy presents with a left-sided scrotal swelling. A scrotal ultrasound reveals a varicocele.

# THEME: SUTURE MATERIALS

**A** Catgut

**B** Monocryl

**C** PDS

**D** Prolene

**E** Silk

**F** Skin clips

**G** Vicryl

**For each of the following situations, choose the most appropriate suture material from the list above. Each option may be used once, more than once or not at all.**

167 An absorbable suture commonly used for bowel anastomosis.

168 Suture most commonly used for vascular anastomosis.

169 Suture used for mass closure of the abdomen.

170 Material commonly used for suturing the mesh to the abdominal wall in hernia repair.

# THEME: ARTERIAL BLOOD GASES

**A**  Compensated metabolic acidosis

**B**  Compensated metabolic alkalosis

**C**  Compensated respiratory acidosis

**D**  Compensated respiratory alkalosis

**E**  Metabolic acidosis

**F**  Metabolic alkalosis

**G**  Respiratory acidosis

**H**  Respiratory alkalosis

For each of the following situations, choose the most appropriate diagnosis from the list above. You may use each option once, more than once or not at all.

171  A 28-year-old woman with acute pancreatitis presents with severe epigastric pain and vomiting. Her blood gases are: pH 7.5; $p_a(O_2)$ 13.9 kPa; $p_a(CO_2)$ 5 kPa; and bicarbonate 33 mmol/l.

172  A 52-year-old diabetic patient attends pre-admission clinic. He appears to be short of breath. His blood gases are: pH 7.31; $p_a(O_2)$ 14.8 kPa; $p_a(CO_2)$ 3 kPa; and bicarbonate 18 mmol/l.

173  A 64-year-old patient in the ICU on her first post op day following an open aortic aneurysm repair. Her blood gases are: pH 7.31; $p_a(O_2)$ 6.6 kPa; $p_a(CO_2)$ 7.25 kPa; and bicarbonate 24 mmol/l.

# THEME: OBSTRUCTIVE JAUNDICE

**A** Acute pancreatitis

**B** Biliary colic

**C** Carcinoma of the pancreas

**D** Cholangiocarcinoma

**E** Cholecystitis

**F** Chronic pancreatitis

**G** Sclerosing cholangitis

**For each of the following scenarios, choose the most likely diagnosis from the list above. Each option may be used once, more than once or not at all.**

174 A 72-year-old woman presents with jaundice and RUQ pain. On examination she has a palpable mass in the RUQ. Ultrasound scan of the abdomen reveals dilated ducts, but no gallstones are seen.

175 A 43-year-old presents with a 2-week history of jaundice and steatorrhoea. He has a long-term history of ulcerative colitis, which is treated currently with azathioprine.

176 A 56-year-old alcoholic presents with jaundice and recurrent episodes of severe epigastric pain radiating to the back. Liver function tests show bilirubin 143 $\mu$mol/l, alkaline phosphatase 750 IU/l, aspartate aminotransferase 378 IU/l, GGT 1106 IU/l. Her amylase is 121 IU/l.

177 A 33-year-old woman presents to casualty with severe RUQ pain. The pain has been coming and going for the past 2 hours. Full blood count, urea and electrolytes and liver function test results are all normal. On the consultant ward round the next morning her pain has gone and she wishes to go home.

## THEME: STAGING OF TUMOURS

**A** Ann Arbor staging

**B** Breslow's staging

**C** Clark's staging

**D** Duke's staging

**E** Gleason's score

**F** Manchester staging

For each of the following scenarios, choose the most appropriate staging score from the list above. Each option may be used once, more than once or not at all.

178 An excised melanoma found to have a maximum depth of invasion of 6 mm.

179 A 24-year-old presents with a palpable lymph node in the anterior triangle of the neck. Fine needle aspiration shows the presence of Reed–Sternberg cells.

180 A 73-year-old man presents with PSA of 17.6. A transrectal ultrasound-guided biopsy is performed.

# QUESTIONS
# PRACTICE PAPER 2

## THEME: GLASGOW COMA SCALE SCORES

**A** 3

**B** 4

**C** 5

**D** 8

**E** 9

**F** 13

**G** 14

**For each of the following scenarios, choose the most appropriate score from the list above. Each option may be used once, more than once or not at all.**

1  You are called to see a patient on the ward. It is now 2 days following his elective surgery. He is making noises, but no actual words. He opens his eyes to speech and withdraws from painful stimuli.

2  A patient is brought into A&E with a head injury. He is not making any sounds or opening his eyes. He extends in response to pain.

3  You arrive for a pre-operative assessment on a patient on the ward. He is sat up in bed, obeys commands to perform a full neurological examination, but answers yes to all questions.

## THEME: DRAINS

**A**  Closed non-suction drain

**B**  Closed suction drain

**C**  Corrugated drain

**D**  No drain required

**E**  Sump drain

**F**  T-tube

**For each of the following situations, choose the most appropriate drain from the list above. Each option may be used once, more than once or not at all.**

4    Bowel anastomosis following uncomplicated elective surgery.

5    Immediately following thyroidectomy.

6    A high-output enteric fistula.

7    A skin flap.

8    An oesophageal perforation.

# THEME: FRACTURE CLASSIFICATIONS

**A** Colton's classification

**B** Garden's classification

**C** Gustilo and Anderson's classification

**D** Mason's classification

**E** Neer's classification

**F** Salter–Harris classification

**G** Weber's classification

**For each of the following scenarios, choose the most appropriate option from the list above. Each option may be used once, more than once or not at all.**

9  An open tibial fracture.

10  A displaced radial head fracture.

11  A fractured distal radius in an 11-year-old child.

12  An intra-capsular fractured neck of femur.

# THEME: LOCAL ANAESTHETICS

**A** Bupivacaine

**B** Bupivacaine and adrenaline

**C** Bupivacaine and lidocaine

**D** Lidocaine

**E** Lidocaine and adrenaline

**F** Prilocaine

**G** Ropivacaine

For each of the following situations, choose the most appropriate option from the list above. Each option may be used once, more than once or not at all.

13  For a digital nerve block to allow suturing of a clean laceration.

14  For Bier's block to manipulate Colles' fracture.

15  For carpal tunnel decompression under local anaesthesia.

16  For post-operative analgesia after Zadik's procedure under a general anaesthetic.

17  For a spinal anaesthetic.

# THEME: TREATMENT OF FRACTURES

**A** Broad arm sling

**B** Intra-medullary nail

**C** Manipulation under anaesthetic

**D** Open reduction and internal fixation

**E** Thomas' splint

**F** Traction

**For each of the following situations, choose the most appropriate treatment option from the list above. Each option may be used once, more than once or not at all.**

18 A closed fracture of the lateral malleolus above the level of the syndesmosis with talar shift.

19 An undisplaced fracture of the radial head in the patient's non-dominant arm.

20 A closed femoral shaft fracture in a patient injured in an RTA who has also sustained fractures of the tibia and fibula on one side, and radius and ulna on the opposite side.

21 An undisplaced clavicle fracture, with no compromise of the overlying skin.

## THEME: THE LIMPING CHILD

**A** Osteomyelitis

**B** Perthes' disease

**C** Septic arthritis

**D** SUFE

**E** Transient synovitis

**F** Tubercular arthritis

For each of the following scenarios, choose the most appropriate option from the list above. Each option may be used once, more than once or not at all.

22 A 6-year-old boy, weighing 15 kg, presents with a few days history of limp. He complains of intermittent right hip and thigh pain, of which he has previously had less severe episodes.

23 A 6-year-old boy presents with left hip and thigh pain for 2 days. He had a recent sore throat which has now resolved. He is apyrexial. On examination internal rotation is decreased. His white cell count is $7 \times 10^9$, erythrocyte sedimentation rate (ESR) is 2 mm/h and C-reactive protein (CRP) is 2 mg/L.

24 A 2-year-old boy with a chest infection is pyrexial and cries on all movements of the right leg.

25 A 14-year-old boy, weighing 70 kg, presents with pain in the right thigh and knee and a decreased range of abduction.

# THEME: FRACTURED NECK OF FEMUR

**A** Austin Moore hemiarthroplasty

**B** Cannulated screws

**C** Dynamic hip screw

**D** Immediate cannulated screws

**E** Thompson's hemiarthroplasty

**F** Total hip replacement

**For each of the following scenarios, choose the most appropriate treatment option from the list above. Each option may be used once, more than once or not at all.**

26  A 75-year-old woman tripped on the pavement and has a displaced subcapital fractured left neck of femur. She also has hypertension and type 2 diabetes.

27  A previously fit and well 60-year-old woman fell downstairs sustaining a minimally displaced subcapital fracture of the left neck of femur.

28  An 82-year-old with a previous history of myocardial infarction fell while walking the dog. He sustains a two-part inter-trochanteric fracture of the right neck of femur.

# THEME: ISCHAEMIC LIMBS

**A**  Amputation

**B**  Angiogram

**C**  Angiogram and bypass

**D**  Angiogram and thrombolysis

**E**  Angioplasty

**F**  Best medical therapy

**G**  Embolectomy

**H**  Intravenous heparin

**For each of the following scenarios, choose the most appropriate option from the list above. Each option may be used once, more than once or not at all.**

29   A patient presents with a history of sudden onset of a painful, cold, numb left foot. There are no previous symptoms. The pulse is irregularly irregular, with no pulses below femoral in left leg and all pulses present in right leg.

30   A patient with congestive cardiac failure (CCF) who is on a medical ward develops a sudden-onset cold, pulseless, numb right foot. Dorsalis pedis and posterior tibial pulses are absent on the right and all pulses are present on left.

31   A diabetic patient who has been on the ward for several weeks for treatment of large infected foot ulcers develops three black toes on the right foot.

# THEME: ABDOMINAL AORTIC ANEURYSMS

**A**  CT scan

**B**  Emergency surgery

**C**  Elective endoluminal repair

**D**  Elective open repair

**E**  Urgent elective repair

**F**  Ultrasound in 6 months

**G**  Ultrasound in 1 year

**For each of the following scenarios, choose the most appropriate option from the list above. Each option may be used once, more than once or not at all.**

32    A patient seen in clinic following an asymptomatic 3.5 cm AAA being discovered during an ultrasound of the renal tract.

33    A patient known to have an AAA, which was 5.3 cm at the previous clinic appointment, has undergone a CT scan. The scan reveals a 5.7 cm infra-renal aneurysm extending from 0.5 cm below the renal arteries into both common iliacs.

34    A patient known to have a AAA is reviewed in clinic for the third time. Ultrasound reveals an increase in size from 4 cm to 4.5 cm.

35    An asymptomatic patient is reviewed in clinic. The ultrasound shows a 5 cm AAA. A scan taken 6 months before showed a 3.7 cm aneurysm.

## THEME: CAROTID ARTERY DISEASE

**A** Best medical therapy

**B** Endarterectomy left side

**C** Endarterectomy right side

**For each of the following scenarios, choose the most appropriate option from the list above. Each option may be used once, more than once or not at all.**

36 A fit and well 76-year-old patient presents with a history of right-sided facial drooping lasting approximately 12 hours, then fully resolving. Duplex scans show a bilateral carotid artery stenosis of 86%.

37 A 73-year-old woman presents with three episodes of amaurosis fugax affecting the right eye during the past 6 months. Duplex scans reveal a bilateral stenosis of 75%.

38 An 87-year-old man presents with an episode of right-sided hemiparesis which fully resolves after 1 week. Duplex scans show a right-sided stenosis of 100% and a left-sided stenosis of 50%.

39 An 82-year-old woman presents with a history of one episode of vertigo and diplopia resolving within 24 hours. Duplex scans show a left-sided stenosis of 60%.

# THEME: PRE-OPERATIVE INVESTIGATIONS

**A** None

**B** FBC

**C** U&E

**D** U&E + FBC

**E** U&E + FBC + random glucose

**F** U&E + FBC + random glucose + amylase

**G** U&E + FBC + LFTs

**H** U&E + random glucose

For each of the following scenarios, choose the minimum acceptable pre-operative investigations needed from the list above. Each option may be used once, more than once or not at all.

40 A 66-year-old man admitted for elective repair of left inguinal hernia. His past medical history includes hypercholesterolaemia and hypertension. He is on diuretics.

41 A 35-year-old man, with a BMI of 31 kg/m², admitted for elective tonsillectomy. There is no significant past medical history.

42 A 30-year-old woman admitted for elective laparoscopy. She has a past medical history of asthma.

43 A 39-year-old woman, admitted as an emergency with severe pain in the right iliac fossa (RIF). She is awaiting appendicectomy and has been on an intravenous infusion for 24 hours. Her past medical history includes epilepsy.

## THEME: PRE-OPERATIVE INVESTIGATIONS

**A**  Chest X-ray

**B**  ECG

**C**  ECG and chest X-ray

**D**  None

**For each of the following scenarios, choose the most appropriate investigation(s) from the list above. Each option may be used once, more than once or not at all.**

44    A 49-year-old woman with hypertension, non-smoker, admitted for elective varicose vein surgery.

45    A 40-year-old man with asthma and ulcerative colitis, non-smoker, admitted for elective knee arthroscopy.

46    A 30-year-old woman, non-smoker, with a large goitre and no significant past medical history admitted for elective thyroidectomy.

# THEME: HEAD INJURIES

**A**  Admission for neurological observations

**B**  Computed tomography (CT) scan

**C**  Home with advice

**D**  Intubation and ventilation

**E**  Referral to neurosurgery

**F**  Skull X-ray

**For each of the following scenarios, choose the most appropriate option from the list above. Each option may be used once, more than once or not at all.**

47  A 50-year-old man falls and bangs his head on a cupboard. He cannot remember the events of the fall, but remembers everything since. He had a loss of consciousness of approximately 30 seconds witnessed by his wife, who lives with him.

48  A 70-year-old man on warfarin for atrial fibrillation trips and falls. There is no loss of consciousness, but he has large laceration over the occiput. He lives with wife.

49  A 30-year-old woman is hit with a metal bar. She has a depressed skull fracture on X-ray. Her Glasgow Coma Scale (GCS) score is 15.

50  A 35-year-old woman has a head injury in an RTA. She remembers the events and did not lose consciousness. Her GCS score is 15 throughout. She has a left haemotympanum on examination.

# THEME: BLOOD GAS ANALYSIS

   **A**  Respiratory alkalosis

   **B**  Respiratory acidosis with compensation

   **C**  Respiratory acidosis without compensation

   **D**  Metabolic alkalosis

   **E**  Metabolic acidosis with compensation

   **F**  Metabolic acidosis without compensation

**For each of the following situations, choose the most appropriate diagnosis from the list above. You may use each option once, more than once or not at all.**

51   pH 7.47; $pa(O_2)$ 12.3 KPa; $pa(CO_2)$ 4.8 kPa; bicarbonate 25 mmol/l; base excess +5 mmol/l.

52   pH 7.31; $pa(O_2)$ 12.7 KPa; $pa(CO_2)$ 3.2 kPa; bicarbonate 19 mmol/l; base excess –7 mmol/l.

53   pH 7.29; $pa(O_2)$ 8.4 KPa; $pa(CO_2)$ 6.7 kPa; bicarbonate 32 mmol/l; base excess –1 mmol/l.

54   pH 7.28; $pa(O_2)$ 13.8 KPa; $pa(CO_2)$ 5.0 kPa; bicarbonate 20 mmol/l; base excess –8 mmol/l.

# THEME: CONSENT

**A**  Doctor can consent for the patient

**B**  Patient can give valid consent

**C**  Patient's refusal is valid and doctor cannot over-ride

**D**  Parents can consent for the patient

**E**  Refusal is not valid and can be overridden

**For each of the following situations, choose the most appropriate option from the list above. Each option may be used once, more than once or not at all.**

55  A 24-year-old nurse presents with testicular torsion. He refuses surgery despite having had the benefits and risks of the procedure explained.

56  A 15-year-old girl whose parents are abroad, requires an emergency appendicectomy. She understands the operation, its benefits and risks.

57  An 86-year-old woman with dementia, Mini-Mental State score 4/10 is admitted with a fractured neck of femur. Her daughter states that she would not have wanted surgery, but there is no advance directive.

58  A 15-year-old boy needs an appendicectomy. His parents refuse the surgery despite hearing the risks and benefits, but the patient gives consent. The patient has five GCSEs.

# THEME: SCROTAL SWELLINGS

**A**  Epididymal cyst
**B**  Epididymo-orchitis
**C**  Gumma
**D**  Hernia
**E**  Hydrocoele
**F**  Spermatocele
**G**  Testicular torsion
**H**  Testicular tumour
**I**  Varicocele

**For each of the following scenarios, choose the most appropriate option from the list above. Each option may be used once, more than once or not at all.**

59  The patient has a right-sided swelling in the scrotum separate from the testis, which you cannot get above. The swelling transmits a cough impulse.

60  The patient has a left-sided swelling and dull ache for 1–2 weeks. The swelling is separate from the testis and transilluminates.

61  The patient has a generalised, non-tender swelling of the left hemiscrotum, which has been gradually increasing in size for 2 months. The testis and epididymis cannot be defined. The swelling transilluminates.

62  A 28-year-old man presents with a 6-hour history of a painful right hemiscrotum. The testis and epididymis can be defined, with a normal lie of the testis, and the epididymis is tender to palpation. The patient has been feeling generally unwell and has had dysuria for 2 days.

63    A 20-year-old man presents with a 2-hour history of severe
      right-sided testicular pain and swelling. The hemiscrotum is very
      tender, with the testis lying normally.

# THEME: TUMOUR MARKERS

**A** Adrenocorticotropic hormone (ACTH)

**B** CA 19–9

**C** CA 125

**D** Calcitonin

**E** Carcinoembryonic antigen (CEA)

**F** $\alpha$-Fetoprotein

**G** $\gamma$-Glutamyl transferase (GGT)

**H** $\beta$-Human chorionic gonadotrophin (hCG)

**I** Lactate dehydrogenase

**J** Prostate-specific antigen (PSA)

**For each of the following malignancies, choose the most appropriate marker from the list above. Each option may be used once, more than once or not at all.**

64  Colorectal carcinoma

65  Breast cancer

66  Ovarian cancer

67  Prostate cancer

68  Choriocarcinoma

69  Small-cell lung cancer

# THEME: CONGENITAL GASTROINTESTINAL ANOMALIES

**A** Duodenal atresia

**B** Exomphalos

**C** Gastroschisis

**D** Hirschsprung's disease

**E** Hypertrophic pyloric stenosis

**F** Meconium ileus

**G** Oesophageal atresia

**H** Small-bowel atresia

**For each of the following scenarios, choose the most likely anomaly from the list above. Each option may be used once, more than once or not at all.**

70 Neonate girl, born at term, presents with uncovered intestine and an ovary protruding through the abdominal wall to the right of the umbilicus, through a defect of approximately 3 cm.

71 A term neonate boy, who has failed to pass meconium, has now developed bilious vomiting and abdominal distension. Per rectal examination reveals a mucus plug, removal of which temporarily relieves the symptoms, but they recur.

72 A neonate girl presents with bilious vomiting and abdominal distension. She passed meconium, but has not opened her bowels since. An abdominal X-ray reveals distended bowel loops with fluid levels.

73 A neonate boy with trisomy 21 presents with bilious vomiting and abdominal distension on day 2. An abdominal X-ray reveals a double gas bubble.

74 A 1-month-old baby boy presents with repeated projectile vomiting of unaltered feed approximately 10 minutes after feeding.

# THEME: TREATMENT OF GROIN HERNIAS

**A**  Conservative

**B**  Elective surgery

**C**  Emergency surgery

**D**  Observation

**E**  Prompt surgery

**F**  Urgent surgery

**For each of the following scenarios, choose the most appropriate option from the list above. Each option may be used once, more than once or not at all.**

75    A 50-year-old woman presents with a mildly tender, irreducible small lump in the right groin below and lateral to the pubic tubercle. She is systemically well.

76    A 20-year-old man presents with a painless, reducible lump in the right groin above and medial to the pubic tubercle, extending into the scrotum, and which can be controlled by occluding the deep inguinal ring.

77    A 30-year-old man with a painless, irreducible lump in the right groin, above and medial to the pubic tubercle.

## THEME: HERNIAS

A   Epigastric hernia

B   Littre's hernia

C   Maydl's hernia

D   Paraumbilical hernia

E   Richter's hernia

F   Spigelian hernia

G   Umbilical hernia

**For each of the following situations, choose the most appropriate option from the list above. Each option may be used once, more than once or not at all.**

78   A hernia protruding through the bands of the internal oblique muscle at the level of the line of Douglas.

79   A hernia through the linea alba, adjacent to the umbilical cicatrix.

80   A hernia containing the strangulated antimesenteric border of the bowel.

81   A hernia containing a strangulated Meckel's diverticulum.

## THEME: TREATMENT OF GALLSTONES

**A**  Elective laparoscopic cholecystectomy

**B**  Elective open cholecystectomy

**C**  ERCP + sphincterotomy

**D**  Low-fat diet

**E**  Urgent cholecystectomy

**For each of the following scenarios, choose the most appropriate treatment option from the list above. Each option may be used once, more than once or not at all.**

82  A 46-year-old woman with renal calculi has a routine ultrasound which reveals three small stones in the gallbladder.

83  A patient admitted three days ago with RUQ pain, vomiting, rigors and a temperature greater than 38 °C, which have failed to settle despite intravenous antibiotics.

84  A 50-year-old man known to have gallstones in the gallbladder, who has had two previous attacks of biliary colic, one requiring hospital admission. He has a past medical history of epilepsy, and a vagotomy and pyloroplasty.

# THEME: CHEST INJURIES

**A** Aortic dissection/disruption

**B** Cardiac tamponade

**C** Diaphragmatic rupture

**D** Flail chest

**E** Haemothorax

**F** Oesophageal injury

**G** Simple pneumothorax

**H** Tension pneumothorax

**I** Tracheobronchial injury

**For each of the following scenarios, choose the most appropriate option from the list above. Each option may be used once, more than once or not at all.**

85 A restrained driver involved in an RTA develops dyspnoea and tachypnoea prior to arrival in A&E. On examination air entry is decreased on the left side of the chest and decreased bowel sounds are audible.

86 A restrained passenger involved in an RTA develops dyspnoea, tachypnoea and tachycardia. On examination chest wall movements are paradoxical.

87 A restrained front seat passenger involved in an RTA in which a car travelling at high speed collided with a wall, was haemodynamically unstable at the scene. Both radial pulses were absent and he went into cardiac arrest at the scene.

88 A restrained backseat passenger involved in an RTA has remained haemodynamically stable, but is tachypnoeic and dyspnoeic. Examination reveals no tracheal deviation, with decreased chest wall expansion, decreased air entry on the left and a dullness to percussion on this side.

89   A restrained driver involved in a high speed impact with a tree
     has stridor, tachypnoea, dyspnoea and subcutaneous
     emphysema.

# THEME: URINARY TRACT CALCULI

A   Conservative management

B   ESWL

C   Flexible ureteroscopy

D   Laparoscopic ureterolithotomy

E   Open surgery

F   Percutaneous nephrolithotomy

**For each of the following situations, choose the most appropriate option from the list above. Each option may be used once, more than once or not at all.**

90   An asymptomatic patient undergoes an ultrasound scan which reveals a 1 cm renal calculus within a cyst.

91   A symptomatic patient with more than 5 mm calculi within the proximal ureter.

92   A patient who has had an episode of left renal colic, now resolved. Ultrasound reveals a 1 cm calculus at the pelvi–ureteric junction.

93   A symptomatic patient with a 1 cm calculus in the lower pole of the right kidney.

## THEME: STERILISATION

**A**  Autoclave

**B**  Dry heat

**C**  Ethylene oxide

**D**  Glutaraldehyde

**E**  Irradiation

**F**  Low-temperature steam and formaldehyde

**For each of the following instruments, choose the most appropriate form of sterilisation from the list above. You may use each option once, more than once or not at all.**

94  Catheters

95  Flexible nasoendoscope

96  Sutures

97  Small McIndoe scissors

# THEME: ABDOMINAL RESECTIONS

A  Abdomino-perineal resection

B  Anterior resection

C  End ileostomy

D  Extended left hemicolectomy

E  Extended right hemicolectomy

F  Hartmann's procedure

G  Left hemicolectomy with primary anastomosis

H  Right hemicolectomy with primary anastomosis

I  Right hemicolectomy with stoma formation

J  Sigmoid colectomy

K  Transverse colectomy

For each of the following situations, choose the most appropriate resection technique from the list above. Each option may be used once, more than once or not at all.

98  A tumour approximately 20 cm distal to the splenic flexure in the descending colon, which is causing obstruction. There is no perforation or metastases.

99  A tumour of the transverse colon 2 cm from the splenic flexure, which is not causing obstruction, with no metastases.

100  A tumour of the ascending colon approximately 15 cm proximal to the hepatic flexure, which is causing obstruction, but there is no perforation or metastases.

101  A non-obstructing tumour of the sigmoid colon without metastases.

102  A tumour approximately 12 cm from the anus. No obstruction and no metastases.

103 A tumour approximately 6 cm from the anus, palpable per rectum. No obstruction and no metastases.

# THEME: TOURNIQUETS

**A** No tourniquet
**B** Simple tourniquet
**C** Tourniquet at 150 mmHg
**D** Tourniquet at 200 mmHg
**E** Tourniquet at 250 mmHg
**F** Tourniquet at 300 mmHg

**For each of the following scenarios, choose the most appropriate tourniquet from the list above. Each option may be used once, more than once or not at all.**

104 A patient with a blood pressure of 150/90 mmHg undergoing Zadik's procedure.

105 A patient with a blood pressure of 140/80 mmHg undergoing fasciectomy for Dupuytren's contracture.

106 A patient with a blood pressure of 150/114 mmHg undergoing knee arthroscopy, who has previously had a femoropopliteal bypass.

# THEME: BIOPSY TECHNIQUES

**A** Brush cytology
**B** Core biopsy
**C** Endoscopic biopsy
**D** Excisional biopsy
**E** Fine needle aspiration cytology
**F** Frozen section
**G** Incisional biopsy

**For each of the following lesions, choose the most appropriate biopsy technique from the list above. Each option may be used once, more than once or not at all.**

107  A lymph node found during Whipple's procedure.

108  A solitary nodule within the thyroid.

109  A suspected basal cell carcinoma.

110  A mass on the bladder wall.

# THEME: PAROTID SWELLINGS

**A**  Acute bacterial sialolithiasis

**B**  Adenocarcinoma

**C**  Adenolymphoma

**D**  Pleomorphic adenoma

**E**  Sarcoidosis

**F**  Sialolithiasis

**G**  Sjögren's syndrome

**H**  Squamous cell carcinoma

**I**  Viral parotitis

**For each of the following scenarios, choose the most appropriate diagnosis from the list above. Each option may be used once, more than once or not at all.**

111  A 47-year-old man presents with a 6-month history of a slowly growing, smooth lesion in the right parotid. All facial movements are normal.

112  A 70-year-old man presents with a painless swelling of the left parotid which he has had for 3 months. He previously had surgery for a right parotid lesion. All facial movements are normal.

113  A 70-year-old man presents with a rapidly growing, painful, hard, left parotid lump, which has been there for one month. The left side of his mouth is drooping. He has previously had radiotherapy to his parathyroids.

114  A 44-year-old man presents with a 6-month history of initially intermittent painful right parotid swelling related to food. The right parotid is now constantly swollen and tender.

115  A 20-year-old man presents with acute-onset bilateral, painful parotid swelling and testicular pain.

## THEME: JOINT INFECTIONS

**A**  Group B streptococcus

**B**  Haemolytic streptococcus

**C**  *Haemophilus influenzae*

**D**  *Neisseria gonorrhoeae*

**E**  *Staphylococcus aureus*

**For each of the following situations, choose the most appropriate option from the list above. Each option may be used once, more than once or not at all.**

116  Septic arthritis in a 2-year-old child.

117  Septic arthritis in a 9-year-old child.

118  Osteomyelitis in a 49-year-old man.

# THEME: SUTURE MATERIALS

**A**   1 PDS (polydioxanone suture)

**B**   1.0 PDS

**C**   1.0 Prolene

**D**   1.0 Vicryl

**E**   3.0 Nylon

**F**   3.0 Prolene

**D**   3.0 Vicryl

**H**   6.0 Prolene

**I**   Steel wire

For each of the following situations, choose the most appropriate suture material from the list above. Each option may be used once, more than once or not at all.

119   Distal sutures for a femoro-distal anastomosis.

120   Abdominal mass closure following laparotomy.

121   Interrupted sutures following Dupuytren's contracture.

122   Sternal closure following bypass surgery.

# THEME: MULTIPLE ENDOCRINE NEOPLASIA

**A**　Gorlin's syndrome

**B**　Sipple's syndrome

**C**　Werner's syndrome

**For each of the following descriptions, choose the most appropriate MEN syndrome from the list above. Each option may be used once, more than once or not at all.**

123　A very tall 20-year-old man with a high, arched palate, large span and long fingers, presenting with a medullary thyroid carcinoma.

124　A 40-year-old woman presents with bilateral phaeochromocytoma. She has a past medical history of medullary thyroid carcinoma.

125　A 50-year-old woman presents with pituitary adenoma and parathyroid hyperplasia. Her mother also had a pituitary adenoma.

126　A 60-year-old man who has multiple mucosal neuromas presents with a medullary thyroid carcinoma.

# THEME: TYPES OF GRAFT

**A**  Allogenic heterotropic graft

**B**  Allogenic orthotopic graft

**C**  Autogenic graft

**D**  Xenogenic heterotropic graft

**E**  Xenogenic orthotopic graft

**For each of the following situations, choose the most appropriate option from the list above. Each option may be used once, more than once or not at all.**

127  A kidney transplant from mother to son.

128  A baboon's heart into a human recipient.

129  A full thickness skin graft.

130  Pancreas from an unrelated human donor to a recipient.

# THEME: UPPER GASTROINTESTINAL HAEMORRHAGE

**A** Aorto-enteric fistula

**B** Duodenal ulcer

**C** Gastric malignancy

**D** Gastric ulcer

**E** Mallory–Weiss tear

**F** Oesophageal varices

**G** Oesophagitis

**H** Vascular malformation

**For each of the following scenarios, choose the most appropriate option from the list above. Each option may be used once, more than once or not at all.**

131 A 80-year-old woman presents with haematemesis. She has had intermittent epigastric pain after food since the past 6 months. She has lost weight – about 3.5 kg (half a stone). She was recently commenced on diclofenac.

132 A 21-year-old student presents with haematemesis. He drank a large amount of alcohol last night and was retching prior to the haematemesis.

133 A 50-year-old man presents with a massive haematemesis. He is haemodynamically unstable. He has clubbing, palmar erythema, gynaecomastia and hepatomegaly.

134 A 30-year-old man presents with haematemesis. He complains of a year-long history of epigastric pain relieved by eating. He is a smoker.

135 A 64-year-old man presents with haematemesis and melaena. He is haemodynamically unstable. He has a previous history of an AAA repair 15 years ago.

## THEME: LOWER GASTROINTESTINAL HAEMORRHAGE

**A** Angiodysplasia

**B** Colorectal cancer

**C** Crohn's disease

**D** Diverticular disease

**E** Haemorrhoids

**F** Infective

**G** Ulcerative colitis

**For each of the following scenarios, choose the most appropriate option from the list above. Each option may be used once, more than once or not at all.**

136 A 40-year-old patient presents with recurrent episodes of fresh bleeding per rectum, with no associated abdominal pain. Fresh blood, but no mass is found on rectal examination. The patient has telangiectasia on the face and mouth. Haemoglobin is 9.2 g/dl (92 g/l) .

137 A 25-year-old woman presents with a 1-month history of worsening intermittent bloody diarrhoea with mucus, associated with crampy abdominal pain. She has lost 3.5 kg (half a stone). There is clubbing of her fingers.

138 A 70-year-old woman presents with a large, fresh rectal bleed. She has no abdominal pain. She gives a history of altered bowel habit and left-sided abdominal pain relieved by defaecation for 1 year. She has not lost any weight.

139 A 75-year-old man presents with a painless rectal bleed. He complains of altered bowel habit and tenesmus for a month, associated with smaller rectal bleeds. He has lost a 1.5 kg (quarter of a stone).

140 A 30-year-old pregnant woman presents with fresh bleeding per rectum, which she has noticed on the toilet paper.

# THEME: TREATMENT OF HAEMORRHOIDS

**A** Conservative management

**B** Injection sclerotherapy

**C** Lord's procedure

**D** Rubber band ligation

**E** Surgical haemorrhoidectomy

**For each of the following scenarios, choose the most appropriate option from the list above. Each option may be used once, more than once or not at all.**

141  A patient with haemorrhoids in the anal canal, which are noted on routine prostate examination.

142  A patient with intermittent bleeding from large piles which prolapse from the anal canal and have to be replaced manually.

143  A patient with intermittent bleeding from piles which lie within the anal canal.

## THEME: FLUIDS

**A**  0 mmol/l

**B**  4 mmol/l

**C**  4.5 mmol/l

**D**  5 mmol/l

**E**  30 mmol/l

**F**  50 mmol/l

**G**  130 mmol/l

**H**  142 mmol/l

**I**  154 mmol/l

**For each of the following statements, choose the most appropriate concentration from the list above. Each option may be used once, more than once or not at all.**

144  The sodium concentration of serum.

145  The sodium concentration of Hartmann's solution.

146  The sodium concentration of Gelofusine.

147  The sodium concentration of 4% dextrose saline.

148  The potassium concentration of Gelofusine.

# THEME: HYPOVOLAEMIC SHOCK

**A** Class I hypovolaemic shock

**B** Class II hypovolaemic shock

**C** Class III hypovolaemic shock

**D** Class IV hypovolaemic shock

**For each of the following scenarios, choose the most appropriate option from the list above. Each option may be used once, more than once or not at all.**

149 An 18-year-old man involved in an RTA has a fractured right femur and open fracture of the left tibia. His pulse is 109 beats/min regular, blood pressure 114/90 mmHg and respiratory rate 25 breaths/min.

150 A 50-year-old man with a bleeding peptic ulcer. His pulse is 98 beats/min, blood pressure 134/72 mmHg and respiratory rate 20 breaths/min.

151 A 30-year-old pregnant woman, with a per vaginal bleed. Her pulse is 138 beats/min, blood pressure 92/70 mmHg, respiratory rate 35 breaths/min.

# THEME: NUTRITIONAL SUPPORT

**A** Jejunostomy

**B** Nasogastric feeding

**C** Nasojejunal feeding

**D** Oral supplementation

**E** Percutaneous endoscopic gastrostomy (PEG) feeding

**F** Total parenteral nutrition (TPN)

**For each of the following patients, choose the most appropriate form of nutritional support from the list above. Each option may be used once, more than once or not at all.**

152  A patient with severe acute pancreatitis.

153  A patient who has had a cerebrovascular incident affecting their swallowing a week ago.

154  A patient undergoing Whipple's procedure.

155  A patient with Crohn's disease affecting the small bowel.

## THEME: THYROID NEOPLASMS

**A** Anaplastic carcinoma

**B** Follicular carcinoma

**C** Malignant lymphoma

**D** Medullary carcinoma

**E** Metastases

**F** Papillary carcinoma

**For each of the following scenarios, choose the most appropriate malignancy from the list above. Each option may be used once, more than once or not at all.**

156 A 35-year-old woman presents with a painless nodule, gradually increasing in size in the left lobe of the thyroid. Histological examination reveals Psammoma bodies.

157 An 83-year-old woman presents with a rapidly growing hard painless lump in the right lobe of the thyroid, associated with dysphagia.

158 A 47-year-old woman presents with a painless lump gradually increasing in size in the left lobe of the thyroid. Her serum calcitonin level is elevated.

# THEME: NIPPLE DISCHARGE

**A** Ductal carcinoma in situ

**B** Duct ectasia

**C** Intra-ductal papilloma

**D** Peri-ductal mastitis

**E** Physiological discharge

**F** Prolactinoma

**For each of the following scenarios, choose the most appropriate diagnosis from the list above. Each option may be used once, more than once or not at all.**

159 A 20-year-old woman with a bloody single-duct discharge and a palpable mass at the areola. No malignant cells are isolated from the discharge.

160 A 31-year-old woman, smoker, with a purulent discharge associated with tenderness.

161 A 62-year-old woman with a bloody single-duct discharge. There is no palpable mass.

162 A 33-year-old multi-parous woman presents with a multi-ductal white discharge, no blood on dipstick. She is being investigated for weight gain and irregular menstruation.

# THEME: SHOULDER PAIN

**A** Acute calcific tendonitis

**B** Acute dislocation

**C** Frozen shoulder

**D** Glenohumeral arthritis

**E** Recurrent dislocation

**F** Referred from cervical spine

**G** Rotator cuff tear

**H** Subacromial impingement

**For each of the following scenarios, choose the most appropriate option from the list above. Each option may be used once, more than once or not at all.**

163 A 25-year-old woman presents with a 12-hour history of rapidly increasing severe right shoulder pain, worst on abduction between 120 and 170 degrees.

164 An 18-year-old rugby player presents with severe left shoulder pain following a direct blow to the shoulder. The left shoulder appears flattened.

165 A 73-year-old man presents three days following a fall with a painful left shoulder. The pain is worse at night and he is unable to lie on that side. Abduction and external rotation are severely decreased, and all movements are painful.

# THEME: ASA GRADING – CLASSIFICATION OF PHYSICAL STATUS

**A** Class 1

**B** Class 2

**C** Class 3

**D** Class 4

**E** Class 5

**For each of the following patients select the most appropriate ASA (American Society of Anesthesiologists) grade. Each option may be used once, more than once or not at all.**

166 A 54-year-old man with chronic renal failure, requiring dialysis. He wants to have a total hip replacement for severe osteoarthritis.

167 A 64-year-old woman with tablet-controlled hypertension for whom a laparoscopic cholecystectomy has been planned.

168 A 34-year-old man ruptures his anterior cruciate ligament (ACL) playing football and needs to have it repaired.

169 A 32-year-old patient with a 10-year history of ulcerative colitis, fully controlled with medication, due to undergo varicose vein stripping of lower limbs.

170 An 18-year-old man due to undergo inguinal hernia repair. He has a history of severe asthma that needed ICU admission in past. He has to use inhalers four times a day, and is admitted to hospital with an acute exacerbation at least twice a year.

# THEME: STAGING OF TRANSITIONAL CELL CARCINOMA OF BLADDER

A $T_{is}$

B $T_1$

C $T_{2a}$

D $T_{2b}$

E $T_{3a}$

F $T_{3b}$

G $T_{4a}$

H $T_{4b}$

**For each of the following scenarios, choose the most appropriate option from the list above. Each option may be used once, more than once or not at all.**

171  A 67-year-old woman presents with a several-month history of painless haematuria. Ultrasound of upper tracts in normal but urine cytological examination is positive for malignant cells. Bimanual examination under general anaesthetic shows that the tumour is fixed to the left lateral side wall.

172  A 70-year-old man presents for 6-monthly surveillance cystoscopy following a diagnosis and resection of transitional cell carcinoma bladder (stage $T_1$) 2 years ago. A suspicious area is seen and TURBT is carried out. Histological examination shows that the tumour breaches the lamina propria and invades the superficial muscle.

## THEME: PANCREATIC TUMOURS

**A** Carcinoma

**B** Cystadenocarcinoma

**C** Cystadenoma

**D** Glucagonoma

**E** Insulinoma

**F** VIP-oma

**G** Zollinger–Ellison tumour

**For each of the following scenarios select the most likely diagnosis from the list above:**

173 A 40-year-old woman presents with a years history of epigastric pain. She is prompted to visit A+E following an episode of melaena. Endoscopy shows multiple peptic ulcers. CT scan shows tumours affecting the pancreas and duodenum.

174 A 28-year-old man is taken to his GP by his partner who says he has been having episodes of behaving strangely associated with altered conciousness. This is particularly a problem when he skips meals. Has a family history of MEN 1 syndrome.

175 A 50-year-old man is found to have a mass on his pancreas as an incidental finding on CT scan carried out for another reason. He is later found to be diabetic. He has no medical problems apart from a persistant eczematous rash on his buttocks which he has had for over a year.

# THEME: POLYPS

**A** Fibroma

**B** Hyperplastic polyp

**C** Inflammatory polyp

**D** Juvenile polyp

**E** Peutz–Jegher's polyp

**F** Tubular adenoma

**G** Villous adenoma

**For each of the descriptions below, select the most likely type of polyp:**

176 The most common polyp found in children. Present as PR bleeding or by prolapsing through anus. Not pre-malignant.

177 Rare colonic tumour which arises from the submucosal layer. May contain muscle or glandular tissue.

178 Most common type of polyp, usually found in the rectum. No evidence that they undergo malignant change.

# THEME: RADIOLOGICAL APPEARANCES

**A** Diverticular disease

**B** Duodenal atresia

**C** Hirschprung disease

**D** Necrotising enterocolitis

**E** Perforated duodenal ulcer

**F** Sigmoid volvulus

**G** Ulcerative colitis

**For each of the X-ray descriptions below, select the most likely diagnosis from the list above.**

179 Distended loop of bowel and 'beak sign' on instant enema

180 Tubular shaped colon and no faecal matter within affected part of bowel

# QUESTIONS
# PRACTICE PAPER 3

## THEME: URINARY TRACT INFECTIONS

**A** *Chlamydia*
**B** *Escherichia coli*
**C** *Klebsiella*
**D** *Mycobacterium tuberculosis*
**E** *Proteus* spp.
**F** *Schistosoma haematobium*
**G** *Streptococcus pneumoniae*

**For each of the following scenarios, choose the most likely pathogen from the list above. Each option may be used once, more than once or not at all.**

1  A 26-year-old woman presents with ureteric colic. A KUB reveals a staghorn calculus in the right kidney.

2  A 32-year-old HIV-positive woman attends clinic with symptoms of recurrent UTIs. Multiple mid-stream urine specimens have been sent by her general practitioner and have only revealed sterile pyuria.

3  A 35-year-old businessman presents with a first episode of frank haematuria. He has just returned from a business trip to Egypt.

## THEME: ANTIBIOTIC USE

    **A**  7-day course of antibiotics

    **B**  Antibiotics for 24 hours

    **C**  No prophylaxis required

    **D**  Single-dose antibiotics

**For each of the following situations, choose the most appropriate option from the list above. You may use each option once, more than once or not at all.**

4    A 24-year-old man is involved in a road traffic accident (RTA). He was the front seat passenger in a car. He has a compound fracture of his right tibia.

5    An 84-year-old diabetic woman has an elective femoral hernia repair. She has had a previous total hip replacement.

6    A 41-year-old woman has fallen off a ladder. She is brought to casualty with a suspected fracture of the base of skull.

7    A 70-year-old diabetic man is to have an abdominal aortic aneurysm (AAA) repair.

# THEME: DYSPHAGIA

**A**  Achalasia

**B**  Barrett's oesophagus

**C**  Chagas' disease

**D**  Diffuse oesophageal spasm

**E**  Gastro-oesophageal reflux disease

**F**  Oesophageal carcinoma

**G**  Pharyngeal pouch

**H**  Scleroderma

**For each of the following scenarios, choose the most likely diagnosis from the list above. Each option may be used once, more than once or not at all.**

8    A 72-year-old heavy smoker presents with dysphagia, retrosternal discomfort and new-onset hoarseness of voice.

9    A 43-year-old man presents with a recurrent sore throat, halitosis and complains of regurgitating undigested food.

10   A 45-year-old woman presents with dysphagia. Barium swallow shows a 'bird's beak' appearance of the lower oesophagus.

# THEME: INCONTINENCE

**A** Bladder instability

**B** Bladder outlet obstruction

**C** Genuine stress incontinence

**D** Neurogenic incontinence

**E** Psychogenic incontinence

**F** Small bladder capacity

**For each of the following scenarios, choose the most likely diagnosis from the list above. Each option may be used once, more than once or not at all.**

11  A 78-year-old man presents with urinary leakage. This occurs on coughing or sneezing. On further questioning, he admits to decreasing urinary flow, increased frequency of micturition, with small volumes passed. In addition he reports symptoms of incomplete emptying.

12  A 43-year-old woman with known multiple sclerosis presents to clinic with urinary incontinence. She has had two children. She passes water every hour, but often does not have the urge to void. She currently wears 8–10 incontinence pads per day.

13  A 21-year-old woman presents with recurrent urinary tract infection. She passes urine every hour, but sometimes has such urgency that she cannot reach the toilet in time to prevent leakage. Flexible cystoscopy reveals interstitial cystitis.

14  A 38-year-old woman presents with urinary incontinence. This occurs on exercising, coughing or sneezing. She has had four children, all vaginal deliveries.

15  A 36-year-old man presents with occasional urinary incontinence. He gives a history of gonorrhoea, which was successfully treated 1 year ago. He has a reduced urinary flow rate, and a post micturition bladder scan reveals a volume of 560 ml.

# THEME: PRE-OPERATIVE INVESTIGATIONS

**A** Electrocardiogram (ECG)

**B** ECG + FBC

**C** ECG + FBC + urea and electrolytes (U&E)

**D** ECG + FBC + U&E + chest X-ray

**E** ECG + FBC + U&E + chest X-ray + lung function tests

**F** ECG + U&E

**G** No investigation required

**For each of the following scenarios, choose the most appropriate minimum acceptable pre-operative investigations needed from the list above. Each option may be used once, more than once or not at all.**

16 A 55-year-old man presents with a distal radius fracture requiring open reduction and internal fixation. He is otherwise fit and well and is not taking any medication. His body mass index (BMI) is 26 kg/m$^2$ and he is a non-smoker.

17 A 31-year-old man attends pre-admission clinic. He is to undergo elective inguinal hernia repair. He has had a recent chest infection but is otherwise fit and well. He is not taking any medication.

18 A 61-year-old man is to undergo total hip replacement. He is otherwise healthy and is a non-smoker.

## THEME: TREATMENT OF ULCERS

**A** Compression bandaging

**B** Debridement

**C** Excision

**D** Revascularisation

**E** Total contact casting

**For each of the following scenarios, choose the most appropriate treatment option from the list above. Each option may be used once, more than once or not at all.**

19  A 38-year-old type 1 diabetic patient presents with a deep ulcer over the head of the first metatarsal. It is painless and on further examination he has decreased sensation in the whole of the foot.

20  A 65-year-old presents with a large circumferential ulcer just above the medial malleolus. She has marked lipodermatosclerosis around the ulcer. Her ankle–brachial pressure index (ABPI) is 0.56.

21  A 71-year-old presents with a large circumferential ulcer over the shin. There is a smaller ulcer over the medial malleolus. The leg has an inverted champagne bottle appearance. A duplex scan shows patent deep veins and good flow in the posterior tibial and dorsalis pedis arteries.

22  A 69-year-old smoker has had a long-standing ulcer on the medial aspect of his right leg. It measures 4 cm in diameter. Recently it has become increasingly friable. The edges are thickened and raised and on further examination he has palpable right inguinal lymph nodes.

23  A 71-year-old heavy smoker attends clinic with a painful, deep punched-out ulcer on the dorsum of his right foot. On inspection he has some hair loss on the right shin compared with the left, and the right leg is cool to touch.

# THEME: SURGICALLY IMPORTANT ORGANISMS

**A** *Acinetobacter*

**B** *Bacteroides fragilis*

**C** *Escherichia coli*

**D** Fusobacteria

**E** *Klebsiella* spp.

**F** *Pseudomonas aeruginosa*

**G** *Staphylococcus aureus*

**H** *Staphylococcus epidermidis*

**For each of the following scenarios, choose the most likely organism from the list above. Each option may be used once, more than once or not at all.**

24 A 34-year-old man has been on the intensive care unit (ICU) for 4 weeks. He has had multiple infections, and is being treated with different antibiotics. He begins to show signs of multi-system infection including meningitis.

25 A 64-year-old man had a knee replacement 2 months ago. He complains of persistent pain, and X-rays appear to show some loosening of the prosthesis. An aspiration of the joint yields a coagulase-negative staphylococcus.

26 A 34-year-old develops severe sepsis 5 days after pan-proctocolectomy for severe ulcerative colitis. Blood cultures reveal an anaerobe which is penicillin resistant.

27 A 19-year-old man attends with a large tonsillar abscess. Bacteriological examination reveals a Gram-negative rod-shaped organism.

28 A 74-year-old with a chronic venous leg ulcer develops an infection within the ulcer. Bacteriologic examination reveals a Gram-negative bacillus.

# THEME: CORD LESIONS

**A**   Anterior cord syndrome

**B**   Brown–Séquard syndrome

**C**   Cauda equina

**D**   Central cord syndrome

**E**   Posterior cord syndrome

**For each of the following scenarios, choose the most likely diagnosis from the list above. Each option may be used once, more than once or not at all.**

29   A 34-year-old man suffers a knife injury to the back. He is unable to move his left lower limb, and is complaining of severe pain from a further stab injury to the left leg. He is insensate to temperature on the right leg.

30   A 37-year-old woman falls from a horse. She describes a hyperextension type injury and is ataxic.

31   A 64-year-old man falls down a flight of stairs. He is unable to move his right lower leg and cannot feel sharp instruments on the right leg. He still is able to feel coarse touch. X-rays reveal a compression fracture of T12.

32   A 76-year-old man walks into the A&E department. He complains of bilateral upper limb weakness after a fall in the morning. Initial cervical spine X-rays show marked degenerative changes.

# THEME: WOUND COVERAGE

**A**  Fasciocutaneous flap

**B**  Full thickness skin graft

**C**  Latissimus dorsi flap

**D**  Rectus abdominis flap

**E**  Split-skin graft

**F**  Tissue expansion

**For each of the following situations, choose the most appropriate action from the list above. Each option may be used once, more than once or not at all.**

33  A 43-year-old woman is diagnosed with carcinoma of the breast. A mastectomy is recommended, and she wishes to undergo simultaneous breast reconstruction. She is a keen sportswoman and particularly enjoys climbing.

34  A 26-year-old man has an open fracture of a lateral malleolus. After initial fixation, there is still a large wound visible. There is healthy muscle under the wound.

## THEME: BENIGN ANO-RECTAL CONDITIONS

**A** DeLorme's procedure

**B** Diltiazem ointment

**C** Haemorrhoidectomy

**D** Incision and drainage

**E** Lidocaine gel

**F** Rubber band ligation

**G** Seton drainage

**H** Steroid enema

**For each of the following scenarios, choose the most appropriate treatment from the list above. Each option may be used once, more than once or not at all.**

35   A 79-year-old woman presents with a prolapsed rectum.

36   A 29-year-old man presents with pain on defaecation and some fresh bleeding. He gives a history of recurrent constipation. There is a skin tag present at the 12 o'clock position. Digital rectal examination is normal but painful, and proctoscopy cannot be performed due to patient discomfort.

37   A 27-year-old woman presents to clinic 2 months after childbirth. She complains of faeces streaked with fresh blood and the feeling of a lump on defaecation.

38   A 43-year-old man complains of itching around the anus. He also admits to anal pain and occasional purulent discharge from the anus. Proctoscopy reveals a fistula beginning at the dentate line, travelling an inter-sphincteric route.

# THEME: TYPES OF CHEST TRAUMA

**A** Aortic rupture

**B** Cardiac tamponade

**C** Diaphragmatic rupture

**D** Haemothorax

**E** Penetrating cardiac injury

**F** Pneumothorax

**G** Pulmonary contusion

**H** Tension pneumothorax

**I** Tracheobronchial tree injury

For each of the following scenarios, choose the most likely diagnosis from the list above. Each option may be used once, more than once or not at all.

39 A 21-year-old is brought to A&E unconscious. He has been involved in an RTA. Primary survey reveals that he is hypotensive and tachycardic, and a chest X-ray reveals a flail chest but no obvious pneumothorax. He has refractory hypotension, with no obvious point of blood loss, hence a laparotomy is organised. He is intubated in the department and has a 4 unit blood transfusion started in the department. As he is being transferred to the operating theatre he goes into cardiac arrest.

40 A 29-year-old has a stab injury to the left side of the chest. Primary survey shows a large left haemothorax which is subsequently drained with a water seal chest drain. After 30 minutes he appears to be in significant distress. On examination he is tachycardic at 120 beats/min and his blood pressure is 90/50 mmHg. He appears to have engorgement of his neck veins and his heart sounds are difficult to hear.

41  A 34-year-old is brought in with a stab wound to the right side of his chest. Primary survey shows a tension pneumothorax. This is initially treated with needle thoracocentesis. A chest drain is inserted. A check X-ray 30 minutes after tube insertion shows the tube to be in a satisfactory position. The patient continues to be in respiratory distress and a repeat chest X-ray after 30 minutes shows a persistent large pneumothorax.

# THEME: PAIN IN THE RIGHT UPPER QUADRANT

**A** Acute pancreatitis

**B** Ascending cholangitis

**C** Biliary colic

**D** Cholecystitis

**E** Chronic pancreatitis

**F** Empyema

**G** Lower lobe pneumonia

**H** Perforated peptic ulcer

**I** Pulmonary embolism

**J** Subphrenic abscess

**For each of the following scenarios, choose the most appropriate option from the list above. Each option may be used once, more than once or not at all.**

42 A 40-year-old presents with intermittent RUQ pain radiating to the back. It is associated with nausea and vomiting. The patient is not obviously jaundiced, but has dark urine. The patient is apyrexial.

43 A 43-year-old man presents with severe RUQ pain radiating to the back. He is visibly jaundiced and complains of chills and rigors. There are calculi in the gallbladder on ultrasound, but none in the common bile duct.

44 A 60-year-old woman with known diverticular disease, who was previously admitted 1 month ago, presents with nausea, weight loss, anaemia, rigors and RUQ pain radiating to the back. She has a raised white cell count.

45 A 30-year-old man presents with severe RUQ pain radiating to the back, associated with vomiting. His amylase is 1520 somogyi u/dL.

46    A 25-year-old man presents with RUQ pain and pyrexia, but no
      rigors. He has a raised white cell count, normal findings on liver
      function tests and normal amylase. Ultrasound scan is normal.

# THEME: SKIN INCISIONS

**A** Lanz's incision

**B** Left paramedian incision

**C** Lower midline incision

**D** Right paramedian incision

**E** Kocher's incision

**F** Pfannenstiel's incision

**G** Rooftop incision

**H** Rutherford–Morrison incision

**I** Upper midline incision

**For each of the following scenarios, choose the most appropriate skin incision from the list above. Each option may be used once, more than once or not at all.**

47   A 60-year-old woman with rheumatoid arthritis presents with sudden-onset upper epigastric pain. She has recently been taking a higher than usual amount of anti–inflammatory medication. On examination she has a rigid abdomen. A chest X-ray shows gas under the diaphragm.

48   A 34-year-old woman is undergoing elective laparoscopic cholecystectomy. It is proving difficult to dissect away from the liver and the decision is made to convert to an open cholecystectomy.

49   A 73-year old presents with a 3-day history of absolute constipation. On examination she has a temperature of 38.4 °C, a rigid abdomen and is in severe pain. A chest X-ray reveals air under the diaphragm.

50   A 17-year-old boy attends with a 1-day history of RIF pain. On examination he has tenderness in the RIF with rebound tenderness and guarding. Rovsing's sign is positive.

## THEME: VENTILATORS

**A** Assisted spontaneous breathing (ASB)

**B** Biphasic positive airway pressure (BIPAP)

**C** Continuous mandatory ventilation (CMV)

**D** Continuous positive airways pressure (CPAP)

**E** High frequency jet ventilation

**F** Positive end expiratory pressure

**G** Synchronous intermittent mandatory ventilation (SIMV)

**For each of the following statements, choose the most appropriate form of ventilation from the list above. Each option may be used once, more than once or not at all.**

51  The form of ventilation used to assist a patient's inspiratory effort. It is used to effectively 'top-up' a patient's own volume of inspired air.

52  The most frequently used form of ventilation in theatre. It can be set to pressure- or volume-controlled mode.

53  The form of ventilation used on spontaneously breathing patients to splint the alveoli and improve respiratory mechanics.

54  The form of ventilation used to help wean patients from ventilators. Breaths are synchronised with the patient's respiratory efforts.

# THEME: SALIVARY GLAND SWELLINGS

**A** Acinic cell carcinoma

**B** Acute bacterial sialadenitis

**C** Acute viral sialadenitis

**D** Frey's syndrome

**E** Mikulicz's syndrome

**F** Pleomorphic adenoma

**G** Sialolithiasis

**H** Sjögren's syndrome

**For each of the following scenarios, choose the most likely diagnosis from the list above. Each option may be used once, more than once or not at all.**

55 A 64-year-old man attends for routine post-operative follow-up following surgery to remove a stone from his parotid gland. He now complains of diffuse facial sweating before meals.

56 A 21-year-old man presents with bilateral tender swellings of his parotid glands along with bilaterally tender testes.

57 A 43-year-old woman with a history of systemic lupus erythematosus (SLE) presents with a severe dry mouth and dry eyes.

58 A 79-year-old woman with recently diagnosed acute lymphocytic leukaemia presents with symmetrical enlargement of all salivary glands, narrowing of her palpebral fissures and a dry mouth.

59 A 59-year-old woman presents with left parotid swelling. It occurs immediately before meals and is exquisitely tender.

# THEME: MANAGEMENT OF CHEST TRAUMA

**A** Application of three-sided occlusive dressing

**B** Cardiopulmonary resuscitation

**C** Close observation

**D** Immediate open thoracotomy

**E** Insertion of chest drain

**F** Needle aspiration

**G** Needle thoracocentesis

**H** Pericardiocentesis

**I** Urgent arteriography

For each of the following scenarios, choose the best therapeutic option from the list above. Each option may be used once, more than once or not at all.

60    A 31-year-old is brought to A&E unconscious. He has been involved in an RTA. He had a right tension pneumothorax which was treated at the scene by needle thoracocentesis. On arrival he has a heart rate of 134 beats/min, a blood pressure of 82/45 mmHg and a respiratory rate of 38 breaths/min. On examination he has absent breath sounds and hyper-resonance on the right side of the chest with tracheal deviation to the left.

61    A 29-year-old man was involved in an RTA. He was the front seat passenger. He is complaining of severe chest pain. On examination he is tachycardic, with a heart rate of 104 beats/min, a respiratory rate of 20 breaths/min and a blood pressure of 140/68 mmHg. On examination he has slightly reduced air entry on the left base, which is also dull to percussion. The trachea is slightly deviated to the right. Chest X-ray shows a small left haemothorax and a widened mediastinum.

62 A 34-year-old is brought in with a stab wound to the right side of his mediastinum. On arrival to the department he is in cardiac arrest. The ECG trace shows pulseless electrical activity.

# THEME: CARCINOGENS

**A** Bronchial carcinoma

**B** Burkitt's lymphoma

**C** Carcinoma of the bladder

**D** Carcinoma of the cervix

**E** Mucosa-associated lymphoid tissue lymphoma (MALT tumour)

**F** Hepatocellular carcinoma

**G** Hodgkin's lymphoma

**H** Oropharyngeal carcinoma

From the list above, choose the malignancy associated with exposure to the substances/organisms listed below. You may use each option once, more than once or not at all.

63   Schistosoma

64   B-naphthylamine

65   Epstein–Barr virus

66   *Helicobacter pylori*

67   Aspergillus infection

68   Betel nuts

# THEME: INOTROPES

**A** Adrenaline

**B** Dobutamine

**C** Dopamine

**D** Isoprenaline

**E** Noradrenaline

**For each of the following statements, choose the most appropriate inotrope from the list above. Each option may be used once, more than once or not at all.**

69 The inotrope which has the greatest bronchodilator effect.

70 The inotrope used in cardiac arrest situations to provoke ventricular fibrillation.

71 The inotrope that in a low dose (less than 4 $\mu$g/kg per min) can be used to increase glomerular filtration rate and sodium excretion.

72 The inotrope that is used in the treatment of shock to increase total peripheral resistance causing increase in both systolic and diastolic blood pressure.

# THEME: SCROTAL SWELLINGS

**A** Epididymo-orchitis

**B** Fournier's gangrene

**C** Hydrocoele

**D** Testicular malignancy

**E** Testicular torsion

**F** Testicular trauma

**G** Torsion of hydatid of Morgagni

**H** Varicocele

**For each of the following scenarios, choose the most likely diagnosis from the list above. Each option may be used once, more than once or not at all.**

73    A 23-year-old man presents with acute scrotal pain. The right testicle is exquisitely tender and is higher than the left. There is some superficial erythema.

74    A 65-year-old man presents with a scrotal swelling. It has recently enlarged, but is painless. Examination reveals a large soft swelling which transilluminates.

75    A 70-year-old diabetic man presents in septic shock. The scrotum is swollen and dusky purple.

# THEME: TRAUMA

**A** Application of hard collar and head restraints

**B** CT scan of the head

**C** Full spinal and neurological assessment

**D** Immobilisation

**E** Intubation

**F** Plain X-rays of the skull

**For each of the following scenarios, choose the most appropriate next step from the list above. Each option may be used once, more than once or not at all.**

76  A 38-year-old man in a hard collar and with head restraints is brought to A&E by the paramedics on a spinal board. He has fallen from a horse. On arrival, he is unconscious and makes no response to painful stimuli. He has a large boggy swelling around his left occiput.

77  A 26-year-old man falls approximately 6 m from a ladder. He has been unable to walk since, complaining of pain in his feet. X-rays requested from triage confirm bilateral calcaneal fractures.

78  A 48-year-old man is brought to A&E following an RTA. He was unconscious at the scene, but on arrival to the department he was fully conscious. He is now talking in a confused manner, opening his eyes in response to pain, and localising to pain.

## THEME: LOCAL ANAESTHETICS

A   5 ml

B   10 ml

C   20 ml

D   30 ml

E   40 ml

F   50 ml

G   60 ml

H   80 ml

What is the maximum volume of each of the local anaesthetic agents given below that can safely be used in a 80 kg man who is otherwise healthy. Each option may be used once, more than once or not at all.

79   Lidocaine 2%.

80   Bupivacaine 0.5%.

81   Bupivacaine 0.25% with 1 in 200, 000 adrenaline.

82   Lidocaine 1% with 1 in 200, 000 adrenaline.

## THEME: PERIPHERAL NERVE INJURY

**A** Axillary nerve

**B** Median nerve

**C** Musculo-cutaneous nerve

**D** Posterior interosseous nerve of the forearm

**E** Radial nerve

**F** Ulnar nerve

**In the following scenarios which is the most likely nerve to be affected? Each option may be used once, more than once or not at all.**

83 A 21-year-old man suffers an anterior dislocation of his right shoulder. Examination after reduction reveals an area of sensory loss around the lateral aspect of the shoulder.

84 A 53-year-old woman falls onto an outstretched hand. X-rays of the elbow reveal a fracture of the radial neck. She has no sensory loss, but has weak extension of the wrist and cannot extend her fingers.

85 A 66-year-old woman falls, fracturing the surgical neck of humerus. Six months after the injury she continues to struggle to abduct her shoulder.

86 An 8-year-old boy has a supra-condylar fracture of the right elbow. After initial K-wire fixation he reattends clinic for routine follow-up. There is hyper-extension of the metacarpophalangeal joints of the ring and little fingers and flexion of the interphalangeal joints.

87 A 23-year-old man has a deep laceration to the anterior aspect of his arm. When seen in A&E there is pulsatile bleeding from the wound and he is unable to flex at the wrist.

# THEME: CHEMOTHERAPY

**A**  Adjuvant chemotherapy

**B**  Neo-adjuvant chemotherapy

**C**  No chemotherapy

**For each of the following scenarios, choose the most appropriate option from the list above. Each option may be used once, more than once or not at all.**

88  A 46-year-old woman presents with a breast lump. After wide local excision and axillary node clearance she is found to have ductal carcinoma in situ with the excision margins clear and no lymph node involvement.

89  A 54-year-old man has a right hemicolectomy. The histopathological report is well differentiated Duke's B carcinoma with vascular invasion.

90  A 42-year-old woman has a cystectomy for squamous cell carcinoma of the bladder. The histopathological report is a poorly differentiated tumour with micrometastases in adjacent lymph nodes. A pre-operative staging CT did not show any evidence of metastasis.

# THEME: DIAGNOSIS OF ENDOCRINE DISORDERS

**A** 24-hour urinary vanillylmandelic acid (VMA)

**B** Dexamethasone suppression test

**C** Plasma aldosterone levels

**D** Radio-immunoassay of 17-hydroxyprogesterone

**E** Serum calcitonin

**F** Short Synacthen test

**G** Vitamin D levels

**For each of the following scenarios, choose the most appropriate investigation from the list above. Each option may be used once, more than once or not at all.**

91 A 36-year-old man presents with a history of intermittent hypertension, anxiety, palpitations, tachycardia and excess sweating. Phaeochromocytoma is suspected.

92 A 46-year-old woman with history of vitiligo and rheumatoid arthritis presents with pigmentation of the buccal mucosa and skin, loss of body hair and postural hypotension suggestive of Addison's disease.

93 A 54-year-old woman presents with hypertension, polyuria and polydipsia. Renal function, blood sugar and calcium levels are all normal. Conn's disease is suspected.

94 A 6-year-old child with short stature, penile enlargement and history of failure to thrive as an infant is suspected of having congenital adrenal hyperplasia.

95 A 24-year-old woman is referred for investigation after developing excessive hair growth and acne, purple striae over the abdomen and central obesity.

# THEME: TERMS USED FOR DISORDERS OF GROWTH AND DIFFERENTIATION

**A** Agenesis

**B** Atrophy

**C** Dysplasia

**D** Hyperplasia

**E** Hypertrophy

**F** Hypoplasia

**G** Metaplasia

**H** Neoplasia

**For each of the following descriptions, choose the most appropriate option from the list above. Each option may be used once, more than once or not at all.**

96  Increased numbers of red blood cells in individuals living at altitude.

97  Weakness, reduced size and function of an arm immobilised for a long period of time.

98  Change of bladder transitional cell epithelium to squamous epithelium following *Schistosoma haematobium* infection.

99  Anencephaly (failure of neural tube development).

# THEME: TREATMENT OF ANAL CONDITIONS

**A** Anal dilatation

**B** Glyceryl trinitrate (GTN) ointment

**C** Incision and drainage

**D** Injection sclerotherapy

**E** Lateral sphincterotomy

**F** Laying open

**G** Seton insertion

**For each of the following scenarios, choose the most appropriate option from the list above. Each option may be used once, more than once or not at all.**

100  A 25-year-old mother of one presents with severe 'unbearable' anal pain, exacerbated by defaecation. She noticed fresh blood on the toilet paper.

101  A 37-year-old man with a history of multiple perianal abscesses presents with perianal soreness and discharge. MRI confirms the presence of a high trans-sphincteric fistula-in-ano.

# THEME: LOWER LIMB NEUROPATHY

**A** Common peroneal nerve

**B** Deep peroneal nerve

**C** Saphenous nerve

**D** Sciatic nerve

**E** Superficial peroneal nerve

**F** Sural nerve

**G** Tibial nerve

**In the following scenarios which is the most likely nerve to be affected? Each option may be used once, more than once or not at all.**

102 A 24-year-old woman had in a below-knee plaster cast for 6 weeks to immobilise a fracture of the distal fibula. On removal of the cast after 6 weeks, she is unable to dorsiflex or evert has no sensation on the dorsum of her foot up to the second interdigital cleft.

103 A 37-year-old woman reattends clinic following treatment of her short saphenous vein varicosities by multiple stab avulsions. She is complaining of numbness along the lateral border of the foot.

104 A 24-year-old man is involved in an RTA. He has a fracture dislocation of the left hip. Following reduction and internal fixation, he is unable to plantarflex or dorsiflex his foot. He has no sensation below the knee except for the medial aspect of his leg and the upper medial calf.

105 A 69-year-old diabetic man complains of numbness around the medial aspect of the leg following femoro-popliteal bypass grafting using a reversed vein graft.

# THEME: MANAGEMENT OF FRACTURED NECK OF FEMUR

A   Closed reduction and cannulated screws

B   Conservative

C   Dynamic hip screw

D   Hemiarthroplasty

E   Open reduction and internal fixation

F   Total hip replacement

**For each of the following scenarios, choose the most appropriate option from the list above. Each option may be used once, more than once or not at all.**

106   A 27-year-old man is involved in an RTA and injures his right hip. An X-ray shows a displaced (Garden's III) subcapital fractured neck of femur.

107   An 82-year-old fit, well and usually mobile woman has a purely mechanical fall at home. She is found lying on floor by a relative 36 hours later. Her left leg is shortened and externally rotated and X-ray confirms a displaced (Garden's IV) subcapital fractured neck of femur.

108   A 69-year-old man fall in the street sustaining a fracture to the left neck of femur. On X-ray this is seen to be a three-part inter-trochanteric fracture with avulsion of the lesser trochanter.

109   A 77-year-old woman trips while shopping sustaining an inter-trochanteric fracture of the left neck of femur. There is 6 cm subtrochanteric extension.

# THEME: CONDITIONS CAUSED BY MICROBES

A   *Candida albicans*

B   *Clostridium difficile*

C   *Clostridium perfringens*

D   *Escherichia coli*

E   *Helicobacter pylori*

F   *Staphylococcus aureus*

G   *Streptococcus faecalis*

H   *Streptococcus pyogenes*

**For each of the following scenarios, choose the most appropriate option from the list above. Each option may be used once, more than once or not at all.**

110   A 42-year-old human immunodeficiency virus (HIV)-positive man with white fluffy patches in the mouth surrounded by painful areas of erythema.

111   A 12-year-old girl with an enlarging hot, tender, erythematous area on her right leg which began as an insect bite.

112   A 42-year-old diabetic woman with dysuria, frequency and offensive-smelling urine.

113   A 66-year-old gentleman who had a recent operation for evacuation of traumatic haematoma of the thigh develops discoloration and swelling at operation site, with crepitus on examination and subcutaneous gas collection visible on X-ray.

114   An 84-year-old woman, treated for 4 weeks with co-amoxiclav (Augmentin) for a respiratory tract infection, develops profuse, offensive-smelling diarrhoea.

115   A 33-year-old man presents to Accident and Emergency (A&E) with severe epigastric pain and signs of peritonism. Erect chest X-ray shows air under the diaphragm.

# THEME: HYPERSENSITIVITY REACTIONS

**A** Type I hypersensitivity reaction
**B** Type II hypersensitivity reaction
**C** Type III hypersensitivity reaction
**D** Type IV hypersensitivity reaction

**For each of the following scenarios, choose the most appropriate option from the list above. Each option may be used once, more than once or not at all.**

116 A 42-year-old woman develops itching, swelling and erythema at the site of the nickel buckle of a new watch.

117 A 15-year-old girl has a streptococcal throat infection, then goes on to develop post-streptococcal glomerulonephritis.

118 A 14-year-old boy develops sneezing and watering of the eyes in the summer months when the pollen count is high.

119 A 44-year-old renal transplant patient develops graft-versus-host disease.

120 A 22-year-old man develops wheezing, rash and swelling of the mouth and tongue after eating a peanut.

121 A baby develops haemolytic disease of the newborn. The mother is rhesus-negative.

# THEME: MANAGEMENT OF VASCULAR DISEASE

**A** Immediate surgery

**B** Medical management (diabetic and blood pressure control, aspirin, statin) and regular follow-up

**C** Prostaglandin infusion

**D** Surgery after further investigation

**For each of the following scenarios, choose the most appropriate option from the list above. Each option may be used once, more than once or not at all.**

122   A 50-year-old man underwent CT scan to exclude injury following an RTA (negative). A 3 cm AAA is an incidental finding.

123   A 60-year-old man, known to have a 4 cm AAA and history of heavy alcohol use, presents with severe central abdominal pain radiating to the back. He is stable on minimal resuscitation.

124   A 70-year-old woman is found to have a right carotid bruit on routine examination. Duplex ultrasound scan shows 50% stenosis. She is asymptomatic.

125   A 79-year-old man who has had multiple transient ischaemic attacks in past few months, undergoes duplex ultrasound of left carotid showing a 70% stenosis.

# THEME: GLASGOW COMA SCALE SCORES

**A** 4

**B** 7

**C** 7

**D** 8

**E** 10

**F** 13

**G** 14

**For each of the following scenarios, choose the most appropriate score from the list above. Each option may be used once, more than once or not at all.**

126  A 25-year-old motorcyclist is involved in a head-on collision with a lorry. On arrival in A&E he is unable to obey commands, but localises to pain and able to speak but appears confused. He only opens his eyes in response to pain only.

127  A 66-year-old man has a fall in the street hitting his head. On initial assessment GCS is 15; however on arrival in A&E he is unable to obey commands and withdraws only from painful stimuli making incomprehensible sounds and not opening his eyes at all.

128  A 44-year-old known IVDU is brought to A&E after being found collapsed after a suspected overdose. He will not open eyes in response to commands but does so in response to painful stimuli. His pupils are pinpoint. His only movement is withdrawal from pain and he doesn't speak.

129  A 29-year-old man involved in a pub brawl is hit over the head with a glass bottle. Able to give a partial history but appears quite confused. He opens his eyes when spoken to and moves on command.

## THEME: MANAGEMENT OF TRANSITIONAL CELL CARCINOMA OF THE BLADDER

**A** Brachytherapy

**B** Cystectomy + reconstruction

**C** Cystectomy + urethrectomy + ileal conduit

**D** Intravesical chemotherapy

**E** MqqqqqqVAC chemotherapy

**F** Nephrectomy

**G** Nephro-urethrectomy

**H** Transurethral resection of bladder tumour (TURBT)

For each of the following scenarios, choose the most appropriate option from the list above. Each option may be used once, more than once or not at all.

130  A 45-year-old woman presents with a 3-week history of haematuria. An IVU reveals a filling defect in the renal pelvis. This is confirmed as a soft-tissue mass on CT scan.

131  A 55-year-old woman is found to have widespread CIS on cystoscopy and biopsy. She is treated initially with several instillations of intravesical BCG. Repeat cystoscopy shows no change in the CIS and urethral biopsy confirms CIS. She is keen for aggressive treatment.

# THEME: HAEMORRHAGIC SHOCK

**A** Class I haemorrhagic shock

**B** Class II haemorrhagic shock

**C** Class III haemorrhagic shock

**D** Class IV haemorrhagic shock

**For each of the following scenarios, choose the most appropriate option from the list above. Each option may be used once, more than once or not at all.**

132 A 20-year-old man involved in an RTA sustains bilateral fractured femurs. He is brought to A&E, where on assessment he is found to be anxious and confused with a pulse rate of 130 beats/min and blood pressure of 70/50 mmHg. Urine output over 1 hour is 10 ml.

133 A 70-year-old patient with a known 5 cm abdominal aortic aneurysm is admitted to A&E with severe central abdominal pain that radiates to the back. Prior to resuscitation, his pulse rate is 110 beats/min, blood pressure 120/100 mmHg and respiratory rate 24 breaths/min. He is slightly anxious but fully lucid.

134 A 60-year-old alcoholic has three episodes of haematemesis (total 500 ml) and melaena. On examination, he is anxious, sweaty and unco-operative with a pulse rate of 126 beats/min, blood pressure 80/60 mmHg and respiratory rate 24 breaths/min.

# THEME: MANAGEMENT OF THYROID DISEASE

**A** Carbimazole

**B** Hemithyroidectomy

**C** Propranolol

**D** Propylthiouracil

**E** Radio-iodide ablation

**F** Subtotal thyroidectomy

**G** Thyroxine

**H** Total thyroidectomy

**For each of the following scenarios, choose the most appropriate management option from the list above. Each option may be used once, more than once or not at all.**

135 A 20-year-old woman presents with a smooth goitre, weight loss, palpitations and diarrhoea. She is diagnosed as having Graves' disease but is unable to tolerate carbimazole due to development of agranulocytosis.

136 A 36-year-old woman is in her second trimester of pregnancy. She was mildly thyrotoxic at first but is increasingly symptomatic and requires treatment.

137 A 56-year-old woman diagnosed with toxic multi-nodular goitre which is unresponsive to medical treatment.

138 A 54-year-old woman presents with a goitre which has been there for a long time but was not bothering her. She is now having some difficulty breathing when lying down and feels 'pressure' in her throat.

# THEME: CAUSES OF JAUNDICE

**A** Carcinoma of head of the pancreas

**B** Gallstones

**C** Gilbert's syndrome

**D** Haemolytic anaemia

**E** Hepatitis

**F** Primary liver carcinoma

**For each of the following scenarios, choose the most appropriate diagnosis from the list above. Each option may be used once, more than once or not at all.**

139 A 20-year-old woman presents with complaints of dark-coloured urine, pale stools and weight loss for a few weeks. On examination she has painless jaundice.

140 A 10-year-old boy with known sickle cell disease presents with pain in the epigastric region. On examination he has jaundice.

141 A known intravenous drug misuser with a history of hepatitis B presents with jaundice and loss of weight. Blood tests reveal raised $\alpha$-fetoprotein. He admits sharing needles with other drug misusers.

## THEME: KNEE INJURIES

**A** Anterior cruciate ligament tear
**B** Lateral meniscus tear
**C** Medial collateral ligament tear
**D** Medial meniscus tear
**E** Patella fracture
**F** Posterior cruciate ligament tear

**For each of the following scenarios, choose the most appropriate option from the list above. Each option may be used once, more than once or not at all.**

142 A 35-year-old rugby player twists his knee during a match. It gradually swells and becomes tender, and he finds himself unable to fully extend it. It is tender over the medial joint line. An X-ray shows evidence of an effusion. Despite aspiration of the traumatic effusion, he is still unable to fully extend the knee.

143 A 25-year-old footballer hyper-extends his knee while attempting to kick the ball. He hears a loud 'popping' sound. The knee swells up immediately. In the following weeks his knee is painful on weight bearing and gives way without warning.

# THEME: TYPES OF ULCER

**A** Arterial ulcer

**B** Curling's ulcer

**C** Marjolin's ulcer

**D** Neuropathic ulcer

**E** Syphilitic ulcer

**F** Venous ulcer

**For each of the following scenarios, choose the most appropriate option from the list above. Each option may be used once, more than once or not at all.**

144 A 64-year-old woman presents with a long-standing ulcer in the gaiter region, which is dressed regularly. The district nurse notices an increase in granulation tissue around the lateral edge which stands proud.

145 A 24-year-old man sustains severe burns during a house fire. He develops epigastric pain and vomits a small amount of blood.

146 A 94-year-old diabetic man develops a painful ulcer with a punched-out appearance over the medial malleolus.

## THEME: TREATMENT OF PROSTATE CANCER

**A**  Androgen ablation

**B**  Brachytherapy

**C**  External beam radiotherapy

**D**  Radical prostatectomy

**E**  Surveillance

**For each of the following scenarios, choose the most appropriate option from the list above. Each option may be used once, more than once or not at all.**

147  An 80-year-old man diagnosed with a $pT_1$ prostate cancer, an incidental finding when the chips obtained from TURP were examined.

148  A 50-year-old man with $pT_2$ prostate cancer diagnosed on rectal biopsy wants curative treatment. He is sexually active and wants to have a minimal chance of developing incontinence and impotence, and wants to reduce the amount of time spent in hospital. He has a small-volume prostate.

149  A 65-year-old man was diagnosed as having prostate cancer with lung and bony metastases and local invasion. He was treated with androgen ablation for 6 months but is now complaining of increasing bony and pelvic pain.

# THEME: MANAGEMENT OF ANKLE INJURIES

**A** Arthrodesis

**B** Closed reduction and plaster of paris

**C** Open reduction and internal fixation

**D** Strict non-weight bearing and physiotherapy only

**E** Support, NSAIDs and early mobilisation

**For each of the following scenarios, choose the most appropriate option from the list above. Each option may be used once, more than once or not at all.**

150  A 46-year-old woman stumbles on a pavement kerb landing awkwardly on her left ankle. She is unable to weight bear. An X-ray shows a fracture of the lateral malleolus only.

151  A 34-year-old footballer has an eversion injury to the right ankle resulting in an avulsion fracture of the medial malleolus. An X-ray also shows an undisplaced fracture of the fibula at the junction between the middle and lower third of the shaft.

152  A 29-year-old woman stumbles while running for the bus, landing heavily on her left ankle. The ankle becomes swollen over the lateral aspect and she has difficulty weight bearing. An X-ray shows no fracture.

## THEME: HAEMORRHOIDS

A  Conservative treatment

B  Evacuation of clot

C  Haemorrhoidectomy

D  Injection sclerotherapy

E  Lord's procedure

F  Rubber band ligation

**For each of the following scenarios, choose the most appropriate option from the list above. Each option may be used once, more than once or not at all.**

153  A 58-year-old man with long-standing constipation presents with rectal bleeding. Colonoscopy reveals normal findings apart from haemorrhoids. The haemorrhoids never prolapse out but over-the-counter topical treatment has failed to offer any relief.

154  A 68-year-old woman has persistently prolapsed piles that are uncomfortable and make anal hygiene difficult.

155  A 29-year-old woman 6 weeks post partum developed haemorrhoids during pregnancy. She presents with a painful irreducible purple perianal swelling and is unable to sit down. Treatment with ice pack and analgesia is unsuccessful.

# THEME: COMPLICATIONS OF COLORECTAL CANCER

**A** Appendicitis

**B** Colocolic intussusception

**C** Fistula formation

**D** Haemorrhage

**E** Invasion into adjacent organ

**F** Obstruction

PAPER 3 QUESTIONS

**For each of the following scenarios, choose the most appropriate option from the list above. Each option may be used once, more than once or not at all.**

156 A 69-year-old man presents with caecal mass presumed to be adenocarcinoma. While undergoing staging investigations, he develops right -sided abdominal pain, guarding and rebound in the RIF associated with fever. There is a mild pyrexia and raised white blood cell count.

157 A 70-year-old man with a known tumour of transverse colon presents with spasms of abdominal pain, abdominal distension and dehydration. A new sausage-shaped mass is palpable in the epigastrium.

158 A 52-year-old man with metastatic adenocarcinoma of the transverse colon presents with faecal vomiting.

# THEME: ABNORMALITIES OF CALCIUM BALANCE

**A** Addison's disease

**B** Hypercalcaemia of malignancy

**C** Hypoparathyroidism

**D** Primary hyperparathyroidism

**E** Secondary hyperparathyroidism

**F** Tertiary hyperparathyroidism

**For each of the following scenarios, choose the most appropriate diagnosis from the list above. Each option may be used once, more than once or not at all.**

159 A 69-year-old woman presents with paraesthesia, muscle cramps and a tingling sensation around the mouth. She has a past history of thyroidectomy for benign goitre.

160 A 54-year-old renal dialysis patient is found to have raised serum calcium and parathyroid hormone (PTH) levels.

161 A 47-year-old woman with a history of postural hypotension and pigmentation of the buccal mucosa and skin is admitted as an emergency with abdominal pain and constipation. She had an episode of renal colic 2 weeks ago.

# THEME: MANAGEMENT OF BENIGN PROSTATIC HYPERPLASIA

**A** Doxazosin

**B** Finasteride

**C** Long-term urethral catheter

**D** Open prostatectomy

**E** Supra-pubic catheter

**F** Transurethral incision of prostate

**G** Transurethral resection of prostate (TURP)

**H** Trial without catheter (TWOC) and $\alpha$-blocker

**I** TWOC alone

**For each of the following scenarios, choose the most appropriate option from the list above. Each option may be used once, more than once or not at all.**

162 A 60-year-old man, day 1 post-op right shoulder hemiarthroplasty for severe arthritis develops acute urinary retention. He is catheterised and found to have a residual volume of 800 ml. Digital rectal examination (DRE) shows a smooth, benign moderately sized prostate.

163 A 65-year-old man has bladder outflow obstruction secondary to benign prostatic hyperplasia (BPH) confirmed by urodynamic studies. Initial success with medical management has been followed by worsening of symptoms, severely affecting his quality of life. DRE reveals a benign-feeling prostate, 50 g in size. Transrectal ultrasound shows no hypoechogenic areas The patient is very fit, well and active and will not accept long-term catheterisation.

164 A 56-year-old man recently remarried and wants to start a family. He has long-standing symptoms of hesitancy, frequency and terminal dribbling. He recently developed occasional haematuria – fully investigated and not found to be due to any other cause than BPH. DRE and ultrasound scan reveal a benign, 40 g prostate.

# THEME: WOUND COMPLICATIONS

**A** Abscess

**B** Delayed healing

**C** Evisceration

**D** Incisional hernia

**E** Superficial infection

**F** Wound dehiscence

**For each of the following scenarios, choose the most appropriate option from the list above. Each option may be used once, more than once or not at all.**

165 A patient who has undergone appendicectomy has the sutures removed, and the medial 2 cm of the wound opens up with only a small serous discharge.

166 A patient who has undergone laparotomy has pink fluid oozing from the wound a day before having the sutures removed. The wound opens and the bowel extrudes.

167 A patient who is 5 days post-op following appendicectomy develops low-grade pyrexia. The wound is full and very tender, and pressure on the medial aspect causes pus to extrude.

## THEME: MANAGEMENT OF HERNIAS

**A**   Conservative management

**B**   Laparoscopic repair

**C**   Mayo's operation 'vest over pants'

**D**   Mesh repair

**E**   Repair via crural (Lockwood) approach

**F**   Repair via high inguinal (Lotheissen) approach

**G**   Resection of bowel, anatomosis and repair of abdominal wall defect

**H**   Shouldice repair

**For each of the following scenarios, choose the most appropriate course of action from the list above. Each option may be used once, more than once or not at all.**

168   A 1-year-old child of African origin has an umbilical hernia since birth. He is asymptomatic.

169   A 38-year-old man presents to outpatients with a femoral hernia which is non-tender and with no evidence of strangulation or obstruction. He wants to have it repaired.

170   A fit and well 32-year-old man develops bilateral inguinal hernias which are increasing in size and becoming unsightly. He has not had any abdominal surgery previously.

# THEME: TREATMENT OF URINARY TRACT INFECTIONS

**A** Aciclovir

**B** Fluconazole

**C** Intravenous co-amoxiclav (Augmentin)

**D** Metronidazole

**E** Mitomycin

**F** Oral ciprofloxacin

**G** Rifampicin

**For each of the following scenarios, choose the most appropriate option from the list above. Each option may be used once, more than once or not at all.**

171 A 24-year-old woman presents with a several-month history of recurrent urinary tract infections (UTIs), recent night sweats and weight loss. Mid-stream urine shows many white blood cells but fails to grow any bacteria. She spent her childhood in Bangladesh.

172 A 47-year-old diabetic woman presents with dysuria, frequency and urgency. Urine is cloudy and smells offensive and is positive for nitrates and leucocytes on urine dipstick. She is systemically well.

173 A 52-year-old man presents to A&E with a two-day history of feeling generally unwell. Over last 12 hours he has developed right loin pain, rigors and has a temperature of 39 °C. Urine dipstick is positive for nitrates.

## THEME: POST-OPERATIVE CRITICAL CARE

**A**  Anaphylactic shock

**B**  Cardiogenic shock

**C**  Hypovolaemic shock

**D**  Neurogenic shock

**E**  Septic shock

**For each of the following scenarios, choose the most appropriate option from the list above. Each option may be used once, more than once or not at all.**

174  A post-operative patient in the ICU has a pulse 112 beats/min, central venous pressure (CVP) 1 mmHg, cardiac output 4 l/min, and stroke volume 50 ml.

175  A post-operative patient in ICU has a pulse 40, CVP 4 mmHg, cardiac output 3 l/min, and stroke volume 80 ml.

176  A post-operative patient in ICU has a pulse 109, CVP 5 mmHg, cardiac output 6 l/min, and stroke volume 40 ml.

## THEME: SKIN LESIONS

**A** Basal cell carcinoma

**B** Bowen's disease

**C** Kaposi's sarcoma

**D** Keratoacanthoma

**E** Lentigo maligna

**F** Malignant melanoma

**G** Seborrhoeic warts

**H** Skin tag

**I** Solar keratosis

**J** Squamous cell carcinoma

**For each of the following scenarios, choose the most likely diagnosis from the list above. Each option may be used once, more than once or not at all.**

177 A 64-year-old man presents with a circumscribed scaly plaque approximately 4 cm diameter on the right calf. Histologic examination shows full thickness epidermal dysplasia.

178 A 52-year-old man presents with an irregularly pigmented plaque on the left cheek, which has been increasing in size and was initially uniformly pigmented.

179 An 84-year-old man presents with an enlarging painless ulcer with everted edges on the back of his neck. It has been bleeding intermittently.

180 A 65-year-old woman presents with a 1-month history of an ulcer over the angle of the mandible with a rolled pearly edge.

# ANSWERS

# ANSWERS
# PRACTICE PAPER 1

## TREATMENT OF TESTICULAR TUMOURS

**1**    A – Chemotherapy

Teratomas are less radiosensitive, and therefore localised disease requires orchidectomy and surveillance. Higher stage disease requires chemotherapy.

**2**    G – Testicular biopsy

Undescended testes have a 20–30-fold greater incidence of developing a tumour. In those who have a previous diagnosis of testicular cancer, the remaining undescended testis should be biopsied.

**3**    B – Chemotherapy and radiotherapy

Seminomas are very radiosensitive. Stage I and II can be treated by orchidectomy and radiotherapy alone, but further spread requires chemotherapy in addition.

# TYPES OF HERNIA

**4**    D – Littre's hernia

A hernia which contains a strangulated Meckel's diverticulum is known as Littre's hernia, and it can progress to gangrene, suppuration and formation of a local fistula.

**5**    B – Femoral hernia

Hernias that present below and lateral to the pubic tubercle are femoral hernias as opposed to inguinal hernias which present above and medial to the pubic tubercle.

**6**    C – Indirect inguinal hernia

Inguinal hernias that can be controlled by pressure over the deep inguinal ring are indirect hernias.

**7**    E – Lumbar hernia

Hernias which appear spontaneously just superior to the iliac crest are most likely to be lumbar hernias. They occur through the lumbar triangle of Petit which is formed by the iliac crest, posterior external oblique and anterior latissimus dorsi.

# BONE TUMOURS

**8    H – Osteosarcoma**

Osteosarcoma has a bimodal distribution with 75% of those affected being aged between 10 and 25 years. The remainder are elderly people with a history of Paget's disease. Osteosarcoma typically presents as a painful mass, most commonly affecting the lower femur and arising from the medullary cavity. It can be a lytic or sclerotic lesion. Those with a history of retinoblastoma have a 5000 times risk of developing an osteosarcoma.

**9    B – Chondrosarcoma**

Chondrosarcomas can present de novo or as malignant transformation of a benign cartilage tumour such an osteochondroma. They usually affect middle-aged or elderly people.

**10    C – Ewing's sarcoma**

Ewing's sarcoma usually affects young people aged between 5 and 15 years. It presents as a lytic lesion which causes a periosteal reaction giving it a characteristic 'onion skin' appearance.

**11    H – Osteosarcoma**

## MANAGEMENT OF ACUTE ISCHAEMIA

### 12     C – Embolectomy

History of limb ischaemia with no previous chronic symptoms, together with a history of atrial fibrillation, is suggestive of an embolus being the cause of the occlusion. As the history is quite short, embolectomy should be carried out.

### 13     A – Amputation

A prolonged history of ischaemia means that reperfusion of the limb is hazardous as this can lead to reperfusion injury, which may result in pulmonary oedema, acute respiratory distress syndrome, renal failure and myocardial dysfunction. In such cases, amputation is often the safest option.

### 14     E – Reconstruction

Acute on chronic ischaemia is usually secondary to thrombus formation on the surface of an atheromatous plaque. If sensory or motor deficit is present and run-off is good, a reconstructive operation is advised.

### 15     A – Amputation

If run-off is poor (with or without thrombus), amputation is recommended. If there is no motor or sensory deficit, thrombolysis is indicated as long as there are no contraindications. If this fails and an angiogram demonstrates poor run-off, amputation should be performed.

# JAUNDICE

## 16    B – Pre-hepatic jaundice

Blood transfusion incompatibility is usually due human error. Antigens in donor blood cause the recipient to produce antibodies against their own red blood cells, resulting in haemolysis of these cells with resulting jaundice.

## 17    C – Post-hepatic jaundice

Complaints of passing pale stools and dark urine when jaundiced is indicative of an obstructive or post-hepatic jaundice. This is due to a lack of production of stercobilinogen which gives the stool a brown colour. Dark urine is also seen in hepatic causes of jaundice and is due to the presence of conjugated (water soluble) bilirubin in the urine.

## 18    B – Pre-hepatic jaundice

Gilbert's syndrome is a type of harmless familial non-haemolytic hyperbilirubinaemia.

## 19    A – Hepatic jaundice

Chlorpromazine is a drug known to cause hepatitis resulting in jaundice.

## NECK LUMPS

### 20    E – Thyroglossal cyst

Thyroglossal cysts are remnants of the thyroglossal duct which runs from the back of the tongue to and including the middle third of the hyoid bone. They are midline structures which can be differentiated from thyroid swellings by the fact they move on protrusion of the tongue.

### 21    B – Cystic hygroma

Cystic hygromas are congenital cystic lymphatic malformations at the root of the neck which transilluminate.

### 22    G – Toxic multi-nodular goitre

Thyroid swellings which feel irregular and are associated with symptoms of hyperthyroidism are not likely to be toxic multi-nodular goitres as thyroid cancers rarely present with toxic symptoms.

### 23    A – Branchial cyst

A lumps appearing between the upper and middle third of the sternocleidomastoid in a 30-year-old is most likely to be a branchial cyst, which originates from the remnant of the second branchial arch. It should be excised before it becomes infected.

### 24    C – Lymph node

A supraclavicular mass together with the symptoms described above is highly suggestive of Virchow's node in association with a gastric carcinoma.

# SURGICAL MANAGEMENT OF INFLAMMATORY BOWEL DISEASE

## 25    D – Proctocolectomy and ileo-anal pouch

Ulcerative colitis is restricted to the large bowel and is always continuous with a diseased rectum. The traditional approach to eliminate all disease and remove the risk of developing a malignancy is a proctocolectomy and ileostomy formation. In younger patient for whom a permanent stoma is unacceptable, an alternative is to form a 'pouch' from the ileum and anastomose this to the dentate line. When the rectum is not involved, a colectomy and ileo-rectal anastomosis avoids a stoma.

## 26    G – Subtotal colectomy + ileostomy + mucous fistula

Emergency surgery in ulcerative colitis, eg to treat a perforation is usually managed with subtotal colectomy, ileostomy and mucous fistula. This leaves an intact rectum and anal sphincter for restorative surgery in the future.

## 27    F – Stricturoplasty

This is a bowel preserving technique where inflammatory strictures are incised longitudinally and then sutured transversely, thus widening the bowel wall.

## 28    C – Ileo-caecal resection

Crohn's disease surgery differs from the management of ulcerative colitis as the purpose is to preserve as much bowel length as possible. Due to its relapsing and remitting nature and tendency to affect any part if the gastrointestinal tract, no surgery can be considered curative.

## 29    A – Colectomy and ileorectal anastomosis

This is used in both Crohn's disease and ulcerative colitis to avoid an ileostomy. 33% of patients have a good result and 33% have a poor result – usually due to recurrent disease.

## SCROTAL SWELLINGS

### 30    F – Hydrocele

A hydrocele is an abnormal collection of fluid within the tunica vaginalis. It can be primary or secondary to a disease process such as infection or carcinoma. It is fluctuant, transilluminable and it is impossibe to feel the testis as a separate structure.

### 31    C – Epididymal cyst

An epididymal cyst is a fluid filled swelling connected with the epididymis which is usually painless. It is fluctuant, transilluminable and felt separate to both the testis and the cord structures. It lies above and slightly behind the testis.

### 32    D – Chronic epididymo-orchitis

Chronic epididymo-orchitis is most commonly due to TB but may also be caused by sarcoidosis and unresolved acute epididymo-orchitis. Usually presents as a painless hard nodule and may be associated with a hydrocele or ulceration and sinus formation on the scrotal skin. It may be treated with standard anti-tuberculosis medication.

### 33    J – Varicocele

A varicocele is 'varicose veins of the spermatic cord' and is due to dilatation of the veins in the pampiniform plexus. It is usually asymptomatic but may cause a dragging, aching pain. It is soft, irregularly shaped and non-transilluminable and disappears on lying down. Sudden appearance of a varicocele in older men should alert to the possibility of retroperitoneal disease.

### 34    G – Inguinoscrotal hernia

Inguino-scrotal hernias are those which descend into the scrotum and are most commonly of the indirect type. They are soft, reducible and non-transilluminable and it is impossible to get above them, although possible to feel the testis as a separate structure. A cough impulse is present.

### 35    B – Encysted hydrocele of cord

An encrusted hydrocele ofthe cord is a fluid filled structure which can lie at any point between the inguinal ring and the upper scrotum. It is fluctuant, transilluminable and it is possible to feel the testis as a separate structure.

## UPPER LIMB FRACTURES

### 36    E – Monteggia's fracture

Monteggia's and Galeazzi's fractures are forearm fractures associated with a dislocation. Monteggia's fracture is a fracture of the upper third of the ulna together with a dislocated radial head, whereas Galeazzi's fracture is a fracture of the shaft of the radius together with a dislocation of the inferior radio-ulnar joint.

### 37    A – Barton's fracture

### 38    F – Smith's fracture

Smith's and Colles' fractures are both extra-articular fractures of the distal radius, but in Smith's fracture there is volar displacement of the distal fragment whereas in Colles' fracture there is dorsal and radial displacement. By definition, Colles' fracture must occur within 2.5 cm of the wrist joint. Barton's fracture is an intra-articular fracture of the distal radius associated with subluxation of the carpus.

### 39    D – Galeazzi's fracture

# STAGING OF COLON CANCER

*Colorectal cancers are staged primarily on the pathological features of the resected specimen using Duke's system. Clinical staging takes account of whether the resection margin is involved. Staging is as follows:*

A – Confined to bowel wall

B – Spread through bowel wall but no nodes involved

C – Lymph node involvement

D – Distant metastases

*Stage D was not included in the original staging but is often used. Stage C is often divided into stage C1 (highest node not involved) and stage C2 (highest node involved). Stage is related to 5 year survival rate.*

**40**    C – Duke's C stage

**41**    C – Duke's C stage

**42**    A – Duke's A stage

# URINARY SYSTEM TRAUMA

## 43    F – Urethrogram

Blood at the urethral meatus is a strong indicator of urethral rupture. In these circumstances, catheterisation is contraindicated. Urethrogram should be performed using water-soluble contrast to demonstrate any leaks and if injury is confirmed, a supra-pubic catheter should be sited. Formal urethral repair should be delayed for 3–6 months.

## 44    E – Surgical exploration

If an injury is sustained to the supra-pubic region and bladder trauma is suspected, a cystogram should be carried out as long as there is no blood at the meatus. Testicular trauma often results in haematoma formation. If this is small with no evidence of testicular rupture, it can be managed conservatively. If the haematoma is large, increasingly painful or there is evidence of testicular rupture, surgical exploration and evacuation of haematoma is required.

## 45    B – CT scan

Renal trauma is most commonly blunt. In penetrating injuries or those due to rib fractures associated injuries should be looked for. All such injuries should be investigated by CT scan or high-dose IVU.

# PREPARATION OF PATIENTS FOR ENDOCRINE SURGERY

**46**    G – Vocal cord examination

Patients due to undergo thyroidectomy require vocal cord examination as there is a risk of nerve damage during the operation. They should also be rendered euthyroid to prevent a 'thyroid storm' occurring when the thyroid is handled.

**47**    E – Thallium technetium scan

Parathyroidectomy should be preceded by a technetium scan. This is because although 80% of primary hyperparathyroidism cases are due to a single adenoma, 10–15% have hyperplasia and 2% have two adenomas. All four parathyroids therefore need to be located, since they can occur in a variety of positions from the hyoid bone to the mediastinum.

**48**    D – Phenoxybenzamine and propranolol

Patients due to undergo adrenalectomy must be thoroughly prepared with $\alpha$- and $\beta$-adrenergic blockade using phenoxybenzamine and propranolol, respectively, as potentially fatal changes in the cardiovascular system can occur under anaesthesia and while handling the tumour.

# MANAGEMENT OF PAEDIATRIC DISORDERS

## 49    F – Ramstedt's pyloromyotomy

The baby has typical presenting features of pyloric stenosis secondary to
hypertrophy of the circular pyloric muscles. Aetiology is unknown. It is
diagnosed by carrying out a test feed and ultrasound scan. Patients should be
adequately hydrated and electrolytes corrected prior to surgery.

## 50    B – Gastrografin enema

The scenario suggests meconium ileus, which is found in 15% of babies with
cystic fibrosis due to highly concentrated meconium which obstructs the
terminal ileum pre-natally. This can be diagnosed pre-natally by ultrasound
scan. Gastrografin enema can be therapeutic in an uncomplicated case due to
its detergent-like effect which loosens the meconium. However, the baby
should also be prepared for laparotomy.

## 51    D – Laparotomy and proceed

The history is typical of intussusception. First-line treatment is hydrostatic or
pneumatic reduction if there no evidence of peritonitis and it is less than 24
hours since onset. However, if recurrent, laparotomy is indicated to identify a
precipitating cause, eg Meckel's diverticulum or a polyp.

## RENAL STONES

### 52   C – PCNL

Stones < 2 cm in the kidney or ureter are generally treated with ESWL. However, this is contraindicated in pregnancy or in patients with AAAs which lie in the blast path. In such patients PCNL is a better option. This is also the preferred option for stones > 2 cm or those > 1 cm in the lower pole region as they have poor clearance rates.

### 53   E – Watch and wait

Stones < 0.5 cm are likely to pass spontaneously unless impacted and so a watch and wait policy is acceptable as long as adequate analgesia is given.

### 54   A – ESWL (see above)

### 55   C – PCNL

Nephrectomy is the preferred option for treatment of renal calculi if the affected kidney has a differential function of < 15% (with normal global renal function). The presence of infection in an upper urinary tract obstructed by stone is dangerous and is an indication for urgent surgical intervention irrespective of the size of the stone.

# MANAGEMENT OF THYROID CANCER

**56**    E – Total thyroidectomy and thyroxine replacement

Papillary carcinoma of the thyroid is often seen in younger patients with a history of irradiation to the neck. Histological examination shows pale, empty-looking nuclei – so called 'Orphan Annie' nuclei. The 10-year survival rate is 90%.

**57**    D – Surgery and external beam radiotherapy

Elderly patients are more likely to develop anaplastic carcinomas, which have a very poor prognosis despite treatment with surgery and radiotherapy.

**58**    E – Total thyroidectomy and thyroxine replacement

Medullary carcinomas of the thyroid are tumours of C-cells which produce calcitonin and are associated with familial MEN syndrome.

**59**    D– Surgery and external beam radiotherapy

Lymphoma of the thyroid is treated in a similar way to anaplastic carcinoma but has better results.

# PRURITUS ANI

## 60    B – Anal fissure

Constipated patients (eg due to opioid-based analgesia) can develop anal fissures – longitudinal tears of the lower half of the anal canal. Although haemorrhoids can also present in this way they are infrequently associated with severe pain unless thrombosed. The pain associated with anal fissures can last for 1–2 hours following defaecation.

## 61    A – Anal carcinoma

Anal carcinoma is more common in homosexuals with a history of anal or genital warts and presents with bleeding, pain, swelling or ulceration and may be associated with enlarged inguinal lymph nodes. Diagnosis should be confirmed with examination under anaesthetic (EUA) and biopsy. Syphilis can present in a similar way but usually as an shallow ulcer (chancre) rather than a mass.

## 62    H – Yeast infection

Steroids and other immunosuppressants are used in the medical management of ulcerative colitis and they predispose patients to developing opportunistic yeast overgrowth (eg *Candida* spp). Candidal infections affecting the skin usually cause areas of erythema with a well-demarcated edge.

## 63    D – Fistula-in-ano

Fistula-in-ano can develop de novo or may be associated with Crohn's disease. There is discharge of pus from the external opening.

# MANAGEMENT OF VENOUS DISEASE OF THE LOWER LIMB

## 64   D – Sapheno-femoral ligation

Superficial varicosities can be treated conservatively with support stockings but if increasingly symptomatic (or if patient wishes for cosmetic reasons) surgery is indicated. Long and short saphenous vein incompetence are treated by sapheno-femoral and sapheno-popliteal ligation, respectively. Branch varicosities can be treated by stab avulsions.

## 65   E – Split-skin graft

Debridement and compression bandaging is the usual first-line treatment for venous ulcers, as long as the ABPI is greater than 0.5. Failure to heal after 12 weeks of this treatment is an indication for split-skin grafting, as are ulcers greater than 10 cm$^2$ in size.

## 66   G – Systemic antibiotics

Infected ulcers should be managed by taking a swab for culture followed by regular cleaning and dressing – topical antibiotics should be avoided. Surrounding cellulitis, however, is an indication for intravenous antibiotics.

## 67   B – Elevation and NSAIDs

Thrombophlebitis is best managed with elevation, NSAIDs and support stockings.

# PAEDIATRIC ORTHOPAEDIC DISORDERS

## 68    D – Perthes' disease

The 'limping child' is a commonly encountered problem and may occur in several conditions. Some clue, however, is given by the age of the child as certain disorders are more likely to present at certain ages. Perthes' disease is the name given to avascular necrosis of the femoral head which is most commonly seen in boys aged 5–7 years. It is a self-limiting condition. The radiological changes are usually well established by the time the child presents.

## 69    F – SUFE

SUFE is a less common condition but also more likely to affect boys, although in an older age group (14–16 years). This condition is usually seen in overweight children who are slow to mature. The epiphysis almost always slips backwards and therefore is only visible on the AP X-ray view if severe – therefore the lateral view is essential.

## 70    C – Irritable hip

Transient synovitis or 'irritable' hip is a common cause of limping in young children but should always be a diagnosis of exclusion. Usually it follows a relatively minor gastrointestinal or respiratory tract infection and resolves spontaneously. It must be differentiated from septic arthritis.

# ABDOMINAL SIGNS

**71** C – Cullen's sign

Pancreatitis may be associated with discoloration or bruising around the umbilicus (Cullen's sign) or flanks (Grey Turner's sign). This is due to haemorrhagic pancreatitis with retroperitoneal spread of blood.

**72** D – Grey Turner's sign

**73** E – Murphy's sign

Murphy's sign is seen in acute cholecystitis and should not be able to be reproduced in the left upper quadrant. It is caused by the downward movement of the inflamed gallbladder onto the examining hand during examination. Boas' sign is also seen in acute cholecystitis.

# ABDOMINAL INCISIONS

## 74    G – Pfannenstiel's incision

Pfannenstiel's incision provides excellent access for gynaecological procedures as well as bladder and prostate operations. It can also be used for bilateral hernia repair. In the emergency setting, eg suspected torted ovarian cyst, a midline incision may be more appropriate.

## 75    E – Midline incision

A perforated duodenal ulcer requires access for oversewing and washout therefore an upper midline incision is appropriate.

## 76    B – Kocher's incision

Kocher's incision is a good incision for cholecystectomy on the left and splenectomy on the right. Laparoscopic cholecystectomy is contraindicated in pregnancy.

## 77    C – Lanz incision

Access for appendicitis can be via a Gridiron or Lanz incision. Lanz's incision is more appropriate in a young woman as it is lower and has a better cosmetic result.

## 78    H – Rooftop incision

Curative surgery for carcinoma of the head of the pancreas usually involves a pancreatico-duodenectomy (Whipple's operation) and is carried out via a rooftop incision.

# FULL BLOOD COUNT

Table 1

|   | Hb | MCV | WBC count | Neutrophils | Eosinophils | Platelets |
|---|-----|-----|-----------|-------------|-------------|-----------|
| A | 10.0 | 120 | 9.0 | 6.0 | 0.1 | 300 |
| B | 7.0 | 80 | 8.0 | 5.0 | 0.2 | 250 |
| C | 6.0 | 60 | 7.0 | 4.0 | 0.1 | 170 |
| D | 13.5 | 90 | 19.0 | 16.0 | 0.1 | 290 |
| E | 22 | 87 | 5.0 | 2.5 | 0.3 | 350 |
| F | 15.0 | 89 | 14.0 | 7.5 | 4.0 | 350 |

## 79  F

Amoebic dysentery along with other parasitic infections results in an eosinophilia. This is also seen with allergic reactions and in asthmatics (type I hypersensitivity reaction).

## 80  A

Alcoholics are prone to developing megaloblastic anaemia (low Hb, high MCV). This occurs when there is defective synthesis of DNA and delayed mitoses, resulting in a nuclear-cytoplasmic asynchrony. It is usually due to Vitamin $B_{12}$ OR folate deficiency.

## 81  D

Chronic corticosteroid use can result in an increased release of neutrophilia from the bone marrow storage pool, causing a neutrophilia.

## 82  C

A person diagnosed with right sided colon cancer has often had the tumour for a while prior to diagnosis, and therefore have probably had longstanding insidious blood loss via the GI tract. This results in iron deficiency, causing a hypochromatic, microcytic anaemia.

**83    B**

Haemolytic anaemias, where there is destruction of circulating red blood cells often results in a normocytic anaemia. In addition, release of bilirubin from red blood cells causes jaundice.

**84    E**

Polycythaemia rubra vera is a myeloproliferative syndrome which causes increased amounts of erythroid precursors with increased red cell mass. Haematocrit and blood viscosity are also raised, therefore increasing the risk of DVT in these individuals.

## GALLSTONE DISEASE

**85    A – Conservative management**

Biliary colic and acute cholecystitis can both present with epigastric or RUQ pain but can be differentiated by the fact that there is an inflammatory component with cholecystitis (pyrexia, raised white cell count). Both should be managed conservatively in the first instance with analgesia, IVI (intravenous infusion) and antibiotics and investigated with ultrasound to confirm the diagnosis.

**86    D – Open cholecystectomy**

Routine cholecystectomy is usually differed for six weeks after an acute episode of cholecystitis. This is normally performed laparoscopically unless contraindicated. However, if the acute episode fails to settle or if there is a complication such as empyema, then open cholestectomy is perfomed during the acute episode.

**87    A – Conservative management**

# SALIVARY GLANDS

**88**  A – Parotid gland

The parotid gland lies behind the mastoid process, styloid process and ramus of the mandible and has the facial nerve, retromandibular vein, external carotid artery and auriculotemporal nerve running through it. The parotid duct pierces the buccinator muscle to drain opposite the second upper molar.

**89**  C – Submandibular gland

The submandibular gland is a mixed salivary gland secreting mucous and serous saliva. Its duct enters the floor of the mouth next to the frenulum of the tongue. The sublinguinal gland lies in front of the anterior border of hyoglossus and medial to genioglossus. It is a mucus secreting gland and is supplied by the lingual artery.

**90**  C – Submandibular gland

See answer to Q89

# MANAGEMENT OF HERNIAS

**91**    D – Urgent hernia repair, ie on an elective list but prioritised over benign conditions

This is a femoral hernia, and as such is likely to strangulate. As there is no evidence of strangulation at present, it does not have to be treated as an emergency, but should be treated as a priority.

**92**    D – Urgent hernia repair, ie on an elective list but prioritised over benign conditions

Inguinal hernias in children do not necessarily cause strangulated bowel, but an incarcerated inguinal hernia is likely to produce testicular ischaemia. Hence it does not have to be repaired as an emergency, as there are no acute problems, but it should be done as an urgency.

**93**    D – Urgent hernia repair, ie on an elective list but prioritised over benign conditions

The short duration of this hernia and the fact that it has become irreducible in such a short time span mean that repairing this hernia should be a priority. Again there are no signs suggestive of strangulation and so an emergency operation is not necessary.

**94**    C – Emergency hernia repair

This hernia is showing signs of strangulation – it is red, hot and irreducible. Irrespective of the patient's medical condition, this hernia requires emergency repair. One option may be to attempt to repair it under local anaesthesia.

**95**    A – Conservative management

This is a small, direct, easily reducible hernia. It is at very low risk of strangulation. It can be treated conservatively as it does not seem to be bothering the patient. This decision can be changed should the hernia enlarge or become symptomatic.

# STATISTICS

**96**    K – 95%

The specificity is the ability to detect that which is truly negative. It is given by the equation:

*Specificity = number of true negatives/(number of true negatives + number of false positives) × 100*

In this case: 76/(76 + 4) × 100 = 76/80 × 100 = 95%.

**97**    I – 80%

The sensitivity is the ability of a test to detect a true positive result. It is given by the equation:

*Sensitivity = number of true positives/(number of true positives + number of false negatives) ×100*

In this case 96/(96 + 24) × 100 = 96/120 × 100 = 80%.

**98**    H – 76%

The NPV is the chance that a condition can be ruled out given a negative result. It is given by the equation:

*NPV = (all negative results without condition/all negatives) × 100*

In this case (100–24)/100 × 100 = 76/100 × 100 = 76%.

**99**    L – 96%

The PPV is the chance that a condition is present if identified by a positive test. It is given by the equation:

*PPV = (all positive results with condition/all positive results) × 100*

In this case (100–4)/100 × 100 = 96/100 × 100 = 96%.

# PANCREATIC TUMOURS

### 100    A – Gastrinoma

Peptic ulceration is a feature of 90% of gastrinomas and 30% of gastrinomas are associated with other endocrine tumours (MEN type 1).

### 101    D – Somatostatinoma

Somatostatinomas are rare tumours derived from pancreatic delta cells. Somatostatin delays gastric emptying and inhibits production of both insulin and glucagons. Clinical features are steatorrhoea, diabetes mellitus and cholelithiasis.

### 102    B – Glucagonoma

Glucagonomas result in secondary diabetes due to the hypersecretion of glucagons. Glucagonomas also result in weight loss due to increased gluconeogenesis and anaemia.

# BREAST INVESTIGATIONS

## 103    F – Ultrasound-guided fine needle aspiration

This lump is likely to be due to thyroid enlargement. To exclude malignant disease it is necessary to take cells for cytological examination from any nodules that may be present in the goitre. The easiest way to ensure cells are taken from a nodule is with ultrasound guidance.

## 104    C – Fine needle aspiration

Even though the lump is clinically and radiologically benign, it is good practice to obtain a cytological diagnosis as part of 'triple assessment'.

## 105    F – Ultrasound-guided fine needle aspiration

This woman has a suspicious area on routine mammography. As the area is impalpable it is not possible to do a fine needle aspiration in clinic, but part of the further investigation of the patient would be an ultrasound scan. Hence a fine needle aspiration should be attempted at the same time.

# INTRAVENOUS FLUIDS

## 106    F – Dextran 70

Dextran 70 expands the plasma volume leading to decreased stasis. It also alters the structure of thrombus to a less organised thrombus, which is supposed to produce smaller, less harmful emboli. However, it is not often used as there is a high risk of anaphylaxis, and it is not as effective as heparin.

## 107    E – Compound sodium lactate solution

Compound sodium lactate (also known as Ringer's lactate or Hartmann's solution) is the fluid of choice for initial resuscitation according to ATLS guidelines.

## 108    E – Compound sodium lactate solution

Compound sodium lactate is the only one of the given fluids to contain potassium. It also contains 130 mmol sodium, 111 mmol chloride and 29 mmol lactate.

## 109    B – 0.9% Sodium chloride solution

0.9% Sodium chloride solution contains 150 mmol sodium; 0.45% sodium chloride solution contains 75 mmol sodium; and 4% dextrose/0.18% sodium chloride contains 30 mmol sodium. Compound sodium lactate contains 131 mmol sodium.

## 110    D – 5% Dextrose solution

Water tends to follow the sodium ions, so any fluid containing sodium is more likely to remain in the intravascular compartment. The dextrose in any solution is rapidly metabolised, therefore it is the same as giving water. This is spread throughout body fluid, ie intracellular and extracellular fluid, hence less remains in the intravascular compartment.

# SPECIFIC TESTS

## 111   C – Lachman's test

Traumatic haemarthrosis is usually caused by ACL rupture, tibial spine avulsion or meniscal tears. The mechanism suggests an ACL injury. Although the pivot shift would also identify a torn ACL, it is not recommended in clinic with an anxious patient as it may be very painful.

## 112   B – Froment's test

Froment's test involves asking the patient to hold a piece of paper between the index finger and an adducted thumb. The clinician pulls the paper away. If an ulnar nerve palsy is present, the patient will be unable to adduct the thumb due to paralysis of adductor pollicis. Instead the thumb will flex at the interphalangeal joint due to the action of flexor pollicis longus, which is supplied by the anterior interosseous branch of the median nerve.

## 113   E – Simmonds' test

The most likely diagnosis in this instance is an Achilles' tendon rupture. Simmonds' test involves asking the patient to kneel facing away from you. Squeezing the calf should produce plantar flexion at the ankle joint. Lack of plantar flexion is indicative of an Achilles' tendon rupture.

# CALCULI

## 114   C – Calcium phosphate

Staghorn calculi form in strongly alkaline urine. They are associated with urinary tract infections with urease-forming bacteria such as proteus. They are composed of magnesium ammonium phosphate with calcium.

## 115   A – Bile pigment stone

Only 10% of gallstones are radio-opaque and these tend to be composed of calcium bilirubinate. They are associated with chronic haemolytic disease causing excess bilirubin release.

## 116   B – Calcium oxalate

Calcium oxalate is the most common substance in urinary tract calculi, accounting for approximately 75% of cases.

# NECK LUMPS

## 117  H – Thyroglossal cyst

A thyroglossal cyst occurs anywhere in the midline of the neck from the base of the tongue to the isthmus of the thyroid gland. It is an embryological remnant of the thyroglossal duct, hence attached to the tongue. As with thyroid swellings it moves with swallowing, but unlike thyroid swellings it also moves upwards on protrusion of the tongue.

## 118  C – Chemodectoma

Chemodectomas or carotid body tumours are tumours of the chemoreceptor tissue in the carotid bodies. They arise in the carotid bifurcation at the level of the hyoid bone. There is sometimes a transmitted pulsation from the adjacent arteries, and compression of the arteries may produce symptoms of transient cerebral ischaemia such as black-outs, transient paralysis or paraesthesia.

## 119  D – Cystic hygroma

Cystic hygromas are collections of clear lymph. The majority present within the first few years of life. They are said to have a 'brilliant translucence' due to the lymph.

## 120  E – Lymph nodes

Fever, sore throat, splenomegaly and petechial type rashes are typical of infectious mononucleosis, making the lumps more than likely to be enlarged lymph nodes.

# TYPES OF ULCER

## 121  C – Cushing's ulcer

Cushing's ulcer is a stress ulcer which occurs secondary to head injury.

## 122  F – Marjolin's ulcer

The recent changes include the increased vascularity of the ulcer and the rolled edges suggest malignant change. A squamous cell carcinoma occurring in a chronic venous ulcer is known as Marjolin's ulcer.

## 123  G – Rodent ulcer

Rodent ulcers (also known as basal cell carcinomas) usually arise on sun-exposed areas of the skin. They classically have raised edges with a pearly white appearance.

## 124  B – Curling's ulcer

Curling's ulcer is a stress ulcer associated with burns.

# SKIN LESIONS

## 125  B – Dermatofibroma

This has all the characteristics of a benign lesion (slow growing, smooth and small). It is a dermatofibroma (also known as histiocytoma). A dermatofibroma usually occurs on a limb in middle-aged people. It starts as a hemispherical lump which flattens into a disc. It is usually covered by normal-looking skin and has no associated features.

## 126  H – Strawberry naevus

Strawberry naevi are present from birth. They are usually sessile hemispheres, but as they grow they can become pedunculated. They are compressible but not pulsatile and most common on the head and neck. They may bleed and become ulcerated if knocked.

## 127  A – Basal cell carcinoma

This is a rodent ulcer or basal cell carcinoma. It is locally invasive, but rarely metastasises. The incidence increases with age as it is related to ultraviolet light exposure. For the same reason it most commonly occurs on the face, above a line drawn from the angle of the mouth to the lobe of the ear. The raised pearly edge is characteristic.

## 128  D – Melanoma

This is a melanoma. By definition there is no benign melanoma and the presence of a brown halo and jaundice indicates metastatic spread. The majority develop in people between 20 and 30 of age, and are more common in Caucasians. They often itch but are rarely painful.

## 129  F – Pyogenic granuloma

Pyogenic granulomas are an overgrowth of granulation tissue that usually form after a minor insult such as a scratch or small cut. They are most common on the hands and face. They grow rapidly but rarely more than 1 cm as they outgrow their blood supply.

## 130  C – Keratoacanthoma

A keratoacanthoma is a self-limiting overgrowth of a hair follicle. The central plug is made up of keratin, and it usually presents as a rapidly growing lump, that may begin to regress by the time the person attends clinic. The lump is generally confined to the skin and mobile over subcutaneous tissue. It may be mistaken for a squamous cell carcinoma due to its rapid growth.

## AIRWAY MANAGEMENT

**131**  H – Single-lumen uncuffed endotracheal tube

The soot in the nasal passages and the respiratory distress suggest a smoke inhalation injury. Early intubation is recommended, and uncuffed tubes are used in children to minimise the chance of tracheal damage.

**132**  B – Double-lumen cuffed endotracheal tube

A general anaesthetic will be required, hence a definitive airway with endotracheal intubation. A double-lumen tube is used in thoracic surgery so that one lung can be deflated, allowing better access to the chest.

**133**  D – Needle cricothyroidotomy

It is likely that there is an airway obstruction, and as this man is in respiratory arrest, urgent intervention is required. Percutaneous tracheostomy is time consuming so needle cricothyroidotomy should be attempted. This is a temporising measure and will allow sufficient ventilation for approximately 30 minutes.

**134**  F – Percutaneous tracheostomy

Tracheostomy reduces the work of breathing, which improves the chances of weaning the patient from mechanical ventilation. It is also better tolerated and leads to a reduction in inotropes or vasopressors.

**135**  G – Single-lumen cuffed endotracheal tube

This man again has evidence of smoke inhalation with his nasal hair singeing. A high respiratory rate and reduced oxygen saturation indicate respiratory distress, and as such he requires endotracheal intubation. A single-lumen cuffed tube is most commonly used.

# COLORECTAL CARCINOMA PROCEDURES

## 136 E – Hartmann's procedure

In the acute setting with a patient who has the potential to become extremely unwell through peritonitis, a quick and safe operation is required. Hartmann's procedure involves forming a colostomy and excising the rectum, oversewing the distal end. There is a possibility of reversal once the patient has sufficiently recovered.

## 137 F – Right hemicolectomy

A right hemicolectomy is performed to excise the tumour and the colon which has the same blood supply from the superior mesenteric artery.

## 138 A – Abdomino-perineal resection

This is a low rectal tumour and for complete excision, it would be hazardous and difficult to maintain the sphincter mechanism. Abdomino-perineal resection is the operation of choice, and in this procedure the colon and rectum are excised from the intra-peritoneal and perineal ends.

## 139 F – Right hemicolectomy

Appendiceal carcinoma is an indication for right hemicolectomy.

## 140 F – Right hemicolectomy

This is a good story of presentation of a caecal tumour. A right hemicolectomy should be performed.

## 141 E – Hartmann's procedure

Although anterior resection is possible, in this instance, with the co-morbidities present, a quick operation is essential and it would be better to avoid anastomoses. Hartmann's procedure is therefore the procedure of choice.

## PROSTATISM

### 142    A – Alfuzosin

This man has acute urinary retention. This is common after major limb arthroplasty, especially after spinal anaesthesia. As the residual urine is not greater than 100 ml, it would be appropriate to try a short course of $\alpha$-blocker and trial without catheter. Although the PSA is raised, this may be due to catheterisation or even the acute urinary retention and is not diagnostic of carcinoma of the prostate.

### 143    G – Zolendronic acid

This man has metastatic spread and a very high PSA despite two attempts at hormonal manipulation. Current guidelines from the British Association of Urological Surgeons suggest the use of zoledronic acid in hormone-escape carcinoma of the prostate with bone metastases.

### 144    F – TURP

There is subjective and objective evidence of continued bladder outflow obstruction despite treatment with both an $\alpha$-blocker and $5\alpha$-reductase inhibitor. Surgery should be considered, with the most common being TURP.

### 145    E – Tolterodine

Although this man has increased frequency, urgency and nocturia, his flow rate is greater than 15 ml/s, making bladder outlet obstruction highly unlikely. Bladder instability is the most likely diagnosis, and this can be treated with an antimuscarinic drug such as tolterodine.

# THE LIMPING CHILD

## 146    E – Septic arthritis

The child is septic, with raised inflammatory markers. The diagnosis is septic arthritis of his right hip and he needs a washout of the hip.

## 147    F – SUFE

SUFE is associated with hypogonadism and is said to occur in short-statured children. It is more common in males. The most common examination finding is restricted internal rotation.

## 148    A – DDH

Common pathologies at this age include septic arthritis, DDH and irritable hip. Although babies are screened for DDH some still present at a later age. It is more common in females, associated with congenital foot abnormalities and breech deliveries along with first-born children and multiple deliveries.

## STERILISATION

**149**  D – Steam sterilisation – 15 minutes at 121 °C

Autoclaving or steam sterilisation is most often used to sterilise surgical instruments. Autoclaves operate at either a cycle of 121 °C for 15 minutes or 134 °C for 3 minutes. This is effective against bacteria, spores and viruses.

**150**  A – Glutaraldehyde 2%

Colonoscopes require fast turnaround times and repeated use. Therefore 2% glutaraldehyde is used as it is cheap, efficient, fast and easy to use.

**151**  C – Irradiation

Single-use items which are commercially produced are usually irradiated for sterilisation. This is effective and efficient for large-scale use.

# TYPES OF SHOCK

### 152 D – Class III haemorrhagic shock

Bilateral femoral fractures can cause a blood loss of around 3000 ml and initial treatment of the patient should centre around fluid resuscitation. Class III shock indicates a volume loss of 1500–2000 ml. Patients are usually extremely agitated, tachycardic with a heart rate of between 120 and 140 beats/min. Both the blood pressure and pulse pressure are reduced and the respiratory rate is increased.

### 153 B – Cardiogenic shock

This man has a raised central venous pressure, increased heart rate and decreased blood pressure. This fits the diagnosis of cardiac tamponade, and this is likely to be a case of cardiogenic shock.

### 154 A – Anaphylactic shock

This man has maintained his blood pressure and pulse for over an hour after injury; therefore significant haemorrhagic shock causing sudden cardiovascular collapse is unlikely. Usual treatment of open fractures consists of tetanus prophylaxis, iodine-impregnated dressings and antibiotics (usually either penicillins or cephalosporins with metronidazole). Any of these may cause an allergic response, and this is the most likely cause of the sudden cardiovascular collapse seen here.

### 155 D – Class II haemorrhagic shock

Patients with Class II shock have a blood loss of between 750 ml and 1500 ml. This manifests itself as tachycardia of between 100 beats/min and 120 beats/min, and a normal systolic blood pressure with a reduced pulse pressure. The respiratory rate is mildly elevated and the patient may be slightly confused or agitated.

## PAEDIATRIC ABDOMINAL DISORDERS

### 156 D – Hirschsprung's disease

This child is constipated, however, the apparent frequency of his episodes, along with Down's is suggestive of Hirschsprung's disease. This is characterised by absence of ganglia in Auerbach's plexus. It is a congenital condition associated with Down's. Children either present as neonates failing to pass meconium or older children with failure to thrive, chronic constipation and a distended abdomen.

### 157 E – Intussusception

Intussusception occurs when a segment of bowel invaginates into an adjoining segment. Children present with abdominal pain, blood on rectal examination and the typical passage of redcurrant jelly-like stools. The majority present between 6 and 9 months of age.

### 158 C – Crohn's disease

Although this boy has RIF pain, it is unlikely to be appendicitis given the 6-week course. Inflammatory bowel disease presents in children in the same way as adults, and Crohn's disease commonly affects the terminal ileum and may present as RIF pain or rectal bleeding.

# CONSENT

## 159 A – Accept wishes for non-treatment

Although this man has a chronic mental health problem, he still retains the capacity to make an informed decision about his treatment. He understands that he is likely to die without surgery and his wishes must be respected. Although you may be able to section him under the Mental Health Act, this only allows for treatment of his mental health problem and not for treating the intra-abdominal perforation.

## 160 C – Proceed to treat without consent of patient

A 13-year-old may be 'Gillick' competent in that if he or she understands the implications and possible complications of treatment, they may consent to that treatment without the express permission of their parents. However, in this instance the child would not be allowed to refuse treatment, as this is not covered by Gillick competence. Parental consent has been obtained, and you can proceed to treat without the consent of the child.

## 161 C – Proceed to treat without consent of patient

This patient has known dementia and so does not have the capacity to make an informed decision with regard to treatment options. To proceed to operative treatment of the fracture would be to act in the patient's best interests.

## 162 A – Accept wishes for non-treatment

A signed, witnessed advance directive must be respected. As such, even though the current situation does not relate to the probable cause for the advance directive, the patient's wishes must be respected.

# UROLOGICAL INVESTIGATIONS

### 163    F – Transrectal ultrasound

A raised PSA (upper limit at this age of around 4.5) and a craggy prostate are suspicious of malignancy. Transrectal ultrasound is the imaging of choice, as CT and MRI have not been shown to reliably demonstrate the prostate. It is also imperative to obtain tissue to confirm the diagnosis and to stage the tumour; this can be attempted at the time of the ultrasound.

### 164    A – Abdominal ultrasound

This man is not producing urine. He has been catheterised adequately, as some urine was obtained, therefore he must be either dehydrated or have bilateral ureteric obstruction. Pelvic lymphadenopathy from metastatic carcinoma of the prostate does cause this, and an urgent ultrasound scan is indicated to see whether there is any hydronephrosis.

### 165    A – Abdominal ultrasound

Trans-abdominal ultrasound is the radiological investigation of choice for frank haematuria as it is safe, non-invasive and good at differentiating solid and cystic masses.

### 166    A – Abdominal ultrasound

The left testicular vein drains into the left renal vein, whereas the right testicular vein drains directly into the inferior vena cava. A left-sided varicocele therefore raises the possibility of a left renal vein thrombus which is commonly caused by left-sided renal tumours. An abdominal ultrasound scan is the first-line investigation.

# SUTURE MATERIALS

## 167  G – Vicryl

Vicryl is an absorbable, braided suture with good knotting properties. This makes it ideal for use in bowel anastomosis. Vicryl is easy to handle and easy to position knots with.

## 168  D – Prolene

Prolene is the most commonly used suture for vascular anastomoses. It is a synthetic, non-absorbable monofilament suture. It causes less tissue reaction and less damage to vascular endothelium. The size of the suture used depends on the size of the vessel.

## 169  C – PDS

PDS is a synthetic, monofilament suture wit a good tensile strength. It is completely absorbed by hydrolysis, which occurs over a period of over 180 days. This makes it ideal for mass closure as it has both the strength and reliability required for mass closure of the abdomen.

## 170  D – Prolene

In this situation a non-absorbable suture is better as it allows for less movement of the mesh once the patient begins mobilising. Again, it is relatively inert which makes it an excellent choice.

## ARTERIAL BLOOD GASES

**171**   F – Metabolic alkalosis

Metabolic alkalosis: there is a raised pH with increased bicarbonate and a normal $p_a(CO_2)$. The normal $p_a(O_2)$ indicates that the respiratory system has not begun to compensate. This situation has arisen due to fluid loss caused by vomiting.

**172**   A – Compensated metabolic acidosis

Compensated metabolic acidosis: the pH is reduced with decreased bicarbonate. The respiratory compensation lowers the $p_a(CO_2)$ and increases the $p_a(O_2)$. This patient has diabetic nephropathy, the chronic nature of which has allowed compensation by the respiratory system.

**173**   G – Respiratory acidosis

Respiratory acidosis: the pH is reduced with a raised $p_a(CO_2)$ and a normal bicarbonate. In this situation over-sedation is a possible cause. Her poor respiratory effort has caused a reduction in her $p_a(O_2)$.

# OBSTRUCTIVE JAUNDICE

## 174  C – Carcinoma of the pancreas

In the presence of jaundice with a palpable gallbladder, the cause of the obstruction is unlikely to be stone disease and more likely to be a malignancy causing the obstruction. In addition the dilatation of the bile ducts with no visible stone disease supports this diagnosis. Ultrasound does not pick up all pancreatic tumours; CT scanning is more sensitive.

## 175  G – Sclerosing cholangitis

The steatorrhoea and jaundice are consistent with obstructive jaundice, and along with a long history of ulcerative colitis, predispose to sclerosing cholangitis.

## 176  F – Chronic pancreatitis

The history is typical of pancreatitis, and the recurrent episodes suggest the chronic nature of the disease. In severe cases of chronic pancreatitis, the serum amylase does not necessarily rise, as the cells producing the amylase are destroyed by the disease process.

## 177  B – Biliary colic

This history is typical of biliary colic. The pain settles as the stone is passed and the obstruction is relieved.

## STAGING OF TUMOURS

### 178    B – Breslow's staging

There are two staging systems for melanomas: Clark's staging is defined by invasion of anatomical layers of the skin, whereas Breslow's staging is based on the depth of invasion. In this instance we only know the depth of invasion, hence Breslow's is used.

### 179    A – Ann Arbor staging

The presence of Reed–Sternberg cells indicates Hodgkin's lymphoma. This is staged using the Ann Arbor staging system.

### 180    E – Gleason's score

Prostate carcinoma is staged using Gleason's scoring system.

# ANSWERS
# PRACTICE PAPER 2

## GLASGOW COMA SCALE SCORES

**1**    E – 9

The patient opens his eyes to speech, but not spontaneously so scores 3. The verbal response of making noises but not words gives him a score of 2, and the motor response of withdrawal from pain gives him a score of 4.

**2**    B – 4

The lack of eye opening and verbal response give the patient a score of 1 in each of these categories. Extension to pain implies a decerebrate response, giving a motor score of 2.

**3**    F – 13

This patient has spontaneous eye opening, giving a score of 4, and is able to cooperate for a full neurological examination giving a score of 6. However, the inappropriate answers to questions give him a verbal score of 3.

## DRAINS

**4     D – No drain required**

Routine drainage is not recommended following uncomplicated bowel anastomosis.

**5     B – Closed suction drain**

A closed suction drain is recommended immediately following thyroidectomy to prevent haematoma formation and airway compromise.

**6     E – Sump drain**

A high-output enteric fistula requires a sump drain to allow both aspiration and irrigation without stimulating further output, and to prevent fistula effluent spilling onto the skin.

**7     B – Closed suction drain**

A skin flap requires a closed suction drain to prevent haematoma formation disrupting the blood supply to the flap.

**8     F – T-tube**

T-tubes can be used for CBD (common bile duct) and for oesophageal perforations to prevent further damage to friable tissues.

# FRACTURE CLASSIFICATIONS

**9**     C – Gustilo and Anderson's classification

Open fractures are classified using Gustilo and Anderson's classification.

**10**     D – Mason's classification

Mason classified radial head fractures.

**11**     F – Salter–Harris classification

A distal radial fracture in a child would extend into the epiphysis and is therefore a growth plate injury. These are classified by the Salter–Harris classification.

**12**     B – Garden's classification

Intra-capsular hip fractures are classified using Garden's classification.

# LOCAL ANAESTHETICS

## 13    D – Lidocaine

Lidocaine without adrenaline is the choice of local anaesthetic as the procedure requires rapid onset of anaesthesia. As it is on a digit, adrenaline must not be used.

## 14    F – Prilocaine

Prilocaine is the most commonly used local anaesthetic for intravenous administration in Bier's blocks.

## 15    C – Bupivacaine and lidocaine

A mixture of bupivacaine and lidocaine is best suited for carpal tunnel surgery as it allows both rapid onset of anaesthesia and longer lasting post-operative analgesia.

## 16    A – Bupivacaine

Bupivacaine alone allows longer duration analgesia once the patient has recovered following a general anaesthetic. Again, adrenaline should not be added as the procedure is on a digit.

## 17    A – Bupivacaine

Bupivacaine without adrenaline can be used in spinal anaesthesia.

# TREATMENT OF FRACTURES

**18**   D – Open reduction and internal fixation

This type of fracture is an unstable injury which requires an anatomical reduction and open reduction and internal fixation is necessary to achieve this.

**19**   A – Broad arm sling

This type of fracture requires treatment only to rest the affected part, and the sling provides relief from the pain.

**20**   B – Intra-medullary nail

This patient has undergone polytrauma, and therefore the fractures need to be treated surgically, so the femoral shaft fracture should be treated with an intramedullary nail, rather than Thomas' splint.

**21**   A – Broad arm sling

An undisplaced clavicle fracture, with no neurovascular or skin complications requires only conservative treatment, and a broad arm sling is the best of the options.

# THE LIMPING CHILD

### 22   B – Perthes' disease

Perthes' disease is the most likely diagnosis as it is more common in boys aged 3–12 years who are small for their age. The pain tends to be vague and they can have had similar previous episodes.

### 23   E – Transient synovitis

Transient synovitis is a diagnosis of exclusion, and it is always important to rule out septic arthritis. In this case the child is systemically well with a recent history of viral illness, and normal bloods, as well as loss of internal rotation, making this diagnosis most likely.

### 24   C – Septic arthritis

Septic arthritis is the most likely cause for this child, as there is a source for haematological spread of infection, the child is systemically unwell and there is pain on all movements.

### 25   D – SUFE

SUFE is more common in boys aged 14–16 years who are overweight. It tends to present with knee pain and causes loss of abduction.

# FRACTURED NECK OF FEMUR

**26**    E – Thompson's hemiarthroplasty

This patient requires a hemiarthroplasty as the fracture is displaced and intra-capsular because avascular necrosis is a significant risk. As the patient does not have significant past medical problems restricting the length of anaesthetic, a cemented (Thompson's) hemiarthroplasty would be the better choice.

**27**    D – Immediate cannulated screws

This patient is under the age of 65 years with no significant co-morbidities and a minimally displaced intra-capsular fracture, so cannulated screws as a surgical emergency are the best choice to preserve the blood supply to the femoral head.

**28**    C – Dynamic hip screw

This is an inter-trochanteric fracture, so the blood supply to the femoral head is not at risk, and a dynamic hip screw is the most suitable treatment.

## ISCHAEMIC LIMBS

### 29    G – Embolectomy

The patient is in atrial fibrillation, which is the most likely cause of the embolus in this previously asymptomatic individual.

### 30    D – Angiogram and thrombolysis

CCF is a known exacerbating condition for thrombus formation, and the patient is likely to have been relatively immobile.

### 31    A – Amputation

This is a picture of a patient with chronic arterial insufficiency and acute deterioration. The disease is distal and there is already extensive skin loss and infection, so bypass is not likely to be an option.

# ABDOMINAL AORTIC ANEURYSMS

**32**   G – Ultrasound in 1 year

Annual surveillance is suitable for aneurysms less than 4 cm.

**33**   D – Elective open repair

The gradual increase in size of this aneurysm necessitates an elective repair in a medically fit patient. This aneurysm is unsuitable for endoluminal repair as it is only 0.5 cm below the renal arteries but needs to be 2 cm below for endoluminal repair.

**34**   F – Ultrasound in 6 months

The aneurysm is asymptomatic and between 4.0 cm and 5.5 cm, so surveillance should be increased to 6-monthly.

**35**   E – Urgent elective repair

This rapid increase in size of greater than 1 cm means that urgent surgery is required.

## CAROTID ARTERY DISEASE

**36**    B – Endarterectomy left side

The symptom of facial drooping occurs on the contralateral side, and a stenosis of greater than 75% warrants surgical intervention.

**37**    C – Endarterectomy right side

Visual loss is a symptom which occurs on the ipsilateral side and therefore the right side is responsible for these symptoms.

**38**    A – Best medical therapy

Hemiparesis is a sign which occurs on the contralateral side, but the stenosis on the right side is 100%. Collateral flow is sufficient as the symptoms resolved, so surgery is not required.

**39**    A – Best medical therapy

The symptoms suggest a source in the vertebrobasilar territory, not the carotid, therefore carotid surgery is not indicated.

# PRE-OPERATIVE INVESTIGATIONS

**40**   E – U&E + FBC + random glucose

This patient is over 65 and is on diuretics, both of which are indications for U&E. FBC is indicated by age over 60, as is random glucose.

**41**   H – U&E + random glucose

U&Es and a random glucose are indicated by the patient's abnormal nutritional state (raised BMI).

**42**   B – FBC

An FBC is indicated in all women. No other blood tests are indicated in adults under 60 years in the absence of a significant past medical history.

**43**   F – U&E + FBC + random glucose + amylase

U&Es are indicated as this patient has been on an intravenous infusion for 24 hours. An FBC, amylase and random glucose are indicated in all emergency patients with abdominal pain.

## PRE-OPERATIVE INVESTIGATIONS

**44**    B – ECG

Past medical history of hypertension is an indication for ECG.

**45**    D – None

The patient is under 60 years of age, therefore neither an ECG nor a chest X-ray can be considered routine investigations. Controlled asthma is not an indication for chest X-ray.

**46**    A – Chest X-ray

A chest X-ray is indicated in this case because of the thyroid enlargement.

# HEAD INJURIES

## 47 C – Home with advice

Post-traumatic amnesia and brief loss of consciousness are not indications for admission, and this patient has someone to accompany him home and observe him.

## 48 A – Admission for neurological observations

This patient requires admission for observation as he is on anticoagulants. Intoxication and clotting abnormalities are also indications for admission.

## 49 E – Referral to neurosurgery

A depressed skull fracture is an indication for a neurosurgical consultation.

## 50 B – CT scan

The left haemotympanum suggests a basal skull fracture, and a CT scan is needed to confirm this diagnosis.

## BLOOD GAS ANALYSIS

**51**    D – Metabolic alkalosis

The pH is increased showing alkalosis. The positive base excess and raised bicarbonate indicate a metabolic cause.

**52**    E – Metabolic acidosis with compensation

The pH is decreased indicating acidosis. The decreased bicarbonate and negative base excess indicate that the cause is metabolic. The decreased $pa(CO_2)$ reveals the respiratory compensation.

**53**    B – Respiratory acidosis with compensation

The pH is decreased indicating acidosis. The raised $pa(CO_2)$ indicates a respiratory cause and the increased bicarbonate with a normal base excess indicates metabolic compensation.

**54**    F – Metabolic acidosis without compensation

The pH is decreased indicating acidosis. The decreased bicarbonate and negative base excess indicate a metabolic cause. The normal $pa(CO_2)$ indicates a lack of respiratory compensation.

## CONSENT

**55**    C – Patient's refusal is valid and doctor cannot over-ride

An adult patient who understands the risks and benefits of the surgery but does not consent cannot be forced to undergo the procedure.

**56**    B – Patient can give valid consent

A patient younger than 16 years of age, who understands the procedure and its risks and benefits, is Gillick competent and can give consent to treatment.

**57**    A – Doctor can consent for the patient

No adult can consent for another adult, therefore the daughter cannot consent for her mother. The decision regarding surgery lies with the doctor.

**58**    B – Patient can give valid consent

A patient under 16 years of age with five GCSEs is likely to be Gillick competent. If the doctor considers him Gillick competent he can consent for himself.

## SCROTAL SWELLINGS

### 59    D – Hernia

Since the swelling cannot be got above and transmits a cough impulse the most likely diagnosis is a hernia.

### 60    A – Epididymal cyst

As the swelling is separate from the testis but not generalised, this suggests it is in the epididymis and transillumination suggests that it is cystic.

### 61    E – Hydrocoele

Swelling that cannot be localised to the testis or epididymis and transilluminates points to a hydrocoele.

### 62    B – Epididymo-orchitis

The epididymis alone being tender, normal lie of the testis, and previous urinary symptoms and systemic symptoms point to epididymo-orchitis rather than torsion in this case.

### 63    G – Testicular torsion

The sudden onset severe pain, and severe testicular tenderness point to torsion. The normal lie of the testis does not rule this out.

# TUMOUR MARKERS

## 64   E – CEA

CEA is a non-specific tumour marker which can be used for colorectal carcinoma.

## 65   E – CEA

CEA can also be used as a marker for breast cancer.

## 66   C – CA 125

CA 125 can be used as a marker for ovarian cancer.

## 67   J – PSA

PSA can be used for prostate cancer.

## 68   H – hCG

$\beta$-hCG can be used for choriocarcinoma.

## 69   A – ACTH

ACTH is secreted by small-cell lung cancers.

# CONGENITAL GASTROINTESTINAL ANOMALIES

## 70    C – Gastroschisis

The intestine protruding to the right of the umbilicus points to the diagnosis of gastroschisis instead of exomphalos. Also in exomphalos the intestine has a membranous covering. The ovaries are more commonly involved in gastroschisis.

## 71    D – Hirschsprung's disease

The failure to pass meconium with bilious vomiting and abdominal distension leads to a diagnosis of meconium ileus or Hirschsprung's. The temporary relief of symptoms by removal of the mucus plug make the diagnosis of Hirschsprung's much more likely.

## 72    H – Small-bowel atresia

That the baby has passed meconium rules out meconium ileus and Hirschsprung's. The X-ray finding of distended bowel points to small-bowel atresia as oppose to duodenal atresia.

## 73    A – Duodenal atresia

The double bubble sign on the abdominal X-ray is a feature of duodenal atresia, as there is a gastric bubble and a second duodenal bubble. This condition is linked to Down's syndrome.

## 74    E – Hypertrophic pyloric stenosis

The fact that the child was healthy for the first month and then developed the projectile vomiting, and that the feed is unaltered point to pyloric stenosis, which is more common in males.

PAPER 2 ANSWERS

# TREATMENT OF GROIN HERNIAS

### 75 F – Urgent surgery

The site of the hernia is that for a femoral hernia. Given that there is a high risk of strangulation (approximately 50%) with femoral hernias, all should be treated with urgent surgery.

### 76 B – Elective surgery

The site of this hernia and that it can be controlled by occluding the deep inguinal ring show it to be an indirect inguinal hernia, which extend into the groin more commonly than other hernias. Asymptomatic indirect inguinal hernias have a low risk of strangulation and therefore surgery can be performed electively.

### 77 E – Prompt surgery

The site of the hernia is that for an inguinal hernia. The fact it is irreducible increases the risk of strangulation, but it is still less than a femoral hernia, so surgery should be performed promptly.

## HERNIAS

**78**    F – Spigelian hernia

**79**    D – Paraumbilical hernia

**80**    E – Richter's hernia

**81**    B – Littre's hernia

An umbilical hernia protrudes through the umbilical cicatrix itself. An epigastric hernia protrudes through the fibres of the linea alba in the epigastric region. In Maydl's hernia a W-shaped loop of bowel is trapped in the hernia with the intervening loop strangulated.

# TREATMENT OF GALLSTONES

## 82   D – Low-fat diet

The patient is asymptomatic, and only a small proportion of asymptomatic calculi actually go on to provoke an attack or require surgery. So prophylactic surgery is not required.

## 83   E – Urgent cholecystectomy

In this case the patient is having an acute attack of cholecystitis and may have an empyema, which has failed to settle with conservative treatment and urgent surgery is required.

## 84   B – Elective open cholecystectomy

This patient has had several attacks of biliary colic, and therefore requires surgery. However, he has had previous upper abdominal surgery so an open procedure is required.

# CHEST INJURIES

## 85    C – Diaphragmatic rupture

The decreased bowel sounds audible in the left side of the chest point to diaphragmatic rupture. This condition is more common on the left, the side on which the driver's seatbelt lies.

## 86    D – Flail chest

The paradoxical chest wall movements are characteristic of flail chest, which is associated with respiratory distress.

## 87    A – Aortic dissection/disruption

The rapid deceleration as a mechanism of injury, coupled with the immediate decompensation and loss of radial pulses prior to arrest in this patient, are signs of aortic dissection. This is an injury that results in death at the scene, usually before the arrival of emergency services.

## 88    E – Haemothorax

The decreased air entry and chest wall expansion suggest a haemothorax or pneumothorax, the lack of tracheal deviation rules out tension pneumothorax, and the dull percussion is a sign of haemothorax.

## 89    I – Tracheobronchial injury

Both the rapid deceleration injury and that the patient has stridor and subcutaneous emphysema point to a rupture of the tracheobronchial tree.

# URINARY TRACT CALCULI

### 90    A – Conservative management

Indications for conservative treatment of renal calculi include calculi less than 5 mm diameter, medullary sponge kidney and calculi within cysts.

### 91    D – Laparoscopic ureterolithotomy

This is a large stone load and location of the calculi would require many treatments with ESWL, whereas laparoscopic ureterolithotomy would allow these to be dealt with in a single procedure.

### 92    B – ESWL

Non-complex calculi with a stone burden of less than 2 cm are amenable to treatment with ESWL.

### 93    C – Flexible ureteroscopy

The lower pole of the kidney is unfavourable anatomy for ESWL.

# STERILISATION

### 94    E – Irradiation

This type of equipment is mass produced and can be sterilised industrially in large batches by irradiation.

### 95    D – Glutaraldehyde

This type of equipment is heat sensitive and requires rapid disinfection between patients in clinic. Glutaraldehyde can rapidly accomplish this.

### 96    C – Ethylene oxide

Sutures are both single use and heat sensitive, and ethylene oxide can provide sterilisation without affecting the suture material.

### 97    B – Dry heat

The fine blades of these scissors are very sensitive to corrosion. Therefore a method of sterilisation which does not involve moisture must be used.

# ABDOMINAL RESECTIONS

*All curative resections for colorectal cancer should take a wide resection and regional lymphatics.*

## 98    F – Hartmann's procedure

In this case there is a left-sided tumour with obstruction, so primary anastomosis is not suitable, therefore Hartmann's procedure is the best option.

## 99    E – Extended right hemicolectomy

The location of this tumour requires greater resection than a standard right hemicolectomy.

## 100    H – Right hemicolectomy with primary anastomosis

Primary anastomosis can often be performed in right-sided obstructing tumours if the small intestine is not distended proximal to the ileo-caecal valve.

## 101    J – Sigmoid colectomy

This sigmoid lesion requires a sigmoid colectomy.

## 102    B – Anterior resection

Non-obstructing high rectal tumours are suitable for anterior resection.

## 103    A – Abdomino-perineal resection

Abdomino-perineal resection is necessary for low rectal tumours, within approximately 8 cm of the anus.

# TOURNIQUETS

### 104    B – Simple tourniquet

This procedure requires only a simple tourniquet, to isolate only the digit being operated on; isolation of the whole limb is not required.

### 105    D – Tourniquet at 200 mmHg

This is a procedure on the upper limb which requires a tourniquet, and in the upper limb, tourniquets should be inflated to 50 mmHg over the systolic blood pressure.

### 106    A – No tourniquet

This is a procedure which would usually require a tourniquet, however, the patient has a past history of peripheral vascular disease, which means a tourniquet cannot be used.

# BIOPSY TECHNIQUES

**107**   F – Frozen section

This situation requires an immediate result during the operation.

**108**   E – Fine needle aspiration cytology

The thyroid is easily accessible, and even though architectural data cannot be gained from this technique, if the result is follicular cells, a lobectomy can be performed.

**109**   D – Excisional biopsy

Excisional biopsies are usually performed for skin lesions.

**110**   C – Endoscopic biopsy

This type of lesion can be accessed with a cystoscope to take a sample for a biopsy.

## PAROTID SWELLINGS

**111** D – Pleomorphic adenoma

Pleomorphic adenomas are more common in men between 40 and 60 years of age. They are slow growing, painless and usually unilateral.

**112** C – Adenolymphoma

Adenolymphomas (Warthin's tumour) are more common in men between 60 and 80 years of age. They are painless. Approximately 10% are bilateral and these are usually asynchronous.

**113** H – Squamous cell carcinoma

Squamous cell carcinomas are more common in men and those who have had prior irradiation. They are rapidly growing and aggressive. They are also painful and tend to affect the facial nerve.

**114** F – Sialolithiasis

Sialolithiasis is more common in middle aged men. It is worse immediately prior to eating when salivation is stimulated.

**115** I – Viral parotitis

Parotitis (mumps) is more common in young patients. It is bilateral and acute, and often associated with orchitis.

# JOINT INFECTIONS

### 116   C – *Haemophilus influenzae*

*Haemophilus influenzae* is three times more common a cause of septic arthritis than *Staphylococcus aureus* in children under 5 years.

### 117   E – *Staphylococcus aureus*

*Staphylococcus aureus* is the most common cause of septic arthritis in children over 5 years.

### 118   E – *Staphylococcus aureus*

*Staphylococcus aureus* is the most common cause of osteomyelitis in children over 5 years and in adults.

## SUTURE MATERIALS

### 119   H – 6.0 Prolene

The distal portion of a femoro-distal anastomosis requires very small sutures. Vascular surgery requires smooth (monofilament), non-absorbable sutures.

### 120   A – 1 PDS

Large, absorbable sutures are required to provide strength for a mass abdominal closure.

### 121   F – 3.0 Prolene

Non-absorbable monofilament suture.

### 122   I – Steel wire

Steel wire is required to provide strength for sternal closure.

# MULTIPLE ENDOCRINE NEOPLASIA

### 123   A – Gorlin's syndrome

The patient has a marfanoid appearance which is associated with type MEN IIB, Gorlin's syndrome.

### 124   B – Sipple's syndrome

Type IIA MEN, Sipple's syndrome, is associated with phaeochromocytoma in 20–50%, and these are commonly bilateral.

### 125   C – Werner's syndrome

Pituitary adenoma and parathyroid hyperplasia are common in MEN type I, Werner's syndrome, which has an autosomal dominant inheritance.

### 126   A – Gorlin's syndrome

Type IIB MEN, Gorlin's syndrome is associated with multiple mucosal neuromas.

# TYPES OF GRAFT

*Allografts are grafts from a member of a species to another of the same species. Autografts are grafts from one site on an individual to another site. Xenografts are grafts from a member of a species to a member of another species. Orthotopic grafts are transplanted to the normal anatomical site in the donor. Heterotopic grafts are transplanted to a different anatomical site.*

**127**    A – Allogenic heterotropic graft

Kidneys are transplanted to a different anatomical location in the recipient.

**128**    E – Xenogenic orthotopic graft

This is a transplant between two species.

**129**    C – Autogenic graft

This transplant is from one site on an individual to another site in the same individual.

**130**    A – Allogenic heterotropic graft

The pancreas is transplanted to a different anatomical location in the recipient.

# UPPER GASTROINTESTINAL HAEMORRHAGE

## 131   D – Gastric ulcer

Gastric ulcer is more common in elderly patients. It is associated with pain brought on by food, and often weight loss secondary to this. It is also associated with NSAID use.

## 132   E – Mallory–Weiss tear

Mallory–Weiss tears are associated with retching prior to the onset of haematemesis and alcohol excess.

## 133   F – Oesophageal varices

The patient has stigmata of liver disease which are associated with variceal haemorrhage, which typically causes large bleeds.

## 134   B – Duodenal ulcer

Duodenal ulcers are more common in young men who smoke and are associated with pain relieved by eating.

## 135   A – Aorto-enteric fistula

Aorto-enteric fistulae are a known late complication following AAA repair.

# LOWER GASTROINTESTINAL HAEMORRHAGE

## 136    A – Angiodysplasia

Recurrent painless episodes of rectal bleeding or a single large bleed can be the presentation of this condition. The telangiectasia point to Osler–Weber–Rendu syndrome, which is associated with angiodysplasia.

## 137    G – Ulcerative colitis

The age of this patient and the presence of mucus accompanying the alteration in bowel habit and crampy pain are features of inflammatory bowel disease. Clubbing is also associated with inflammatory bowel disease. Bleeding is more common in ulcerative colitis.

## 138    D – Diverticular disease

Diverticular disease is common in patients over 60, and its incidence increases with age. The length of the history with no associated weight loss and the left-sided pain relieved by defaecation make the diagnosis of diverticular disease more likely than that of colorectal cancer.

## 139    B – Colorectal cancer

This patient has lost weight over a very short period of time, coupled with an alteration in bowel habit and rectal bleeding. These are all sinister features suggesting malignancy.

## 140    E – Haemorrhoids

Haemorrhoids are more common in pregnancy and associated with fresh blood on the toilet paper, and not mixed with stool.

# TREATMENT OF HAEMORRHOIDS

### 141 A – Conservative management

Asymptomatic haemorrhoids do not require treatment.

### 142 D – Rubber band ligation

For large, second-degree haemorrhoids multiple injection sclerotherapy treatments may be required; rubber band ligation offers a better chance of a single treatment.

### 143 B – Injection sclerotherapy

Injection sclerotherapy can be used for symptomatic, first- and second-degree haemorrhoids.

# FLUIDS

**144**  H – 142 mmol/l

**145**  G – 130 mmol/l

**146**  I – 154 mmol/l

**147**  E – 30 mmol/l

**148**  A – 0 mmol/l

The concentrations are shown in the table below.

**Table 3**

| Fluid | Sodium concentration (mmol/l) | Potassium concentration (mmol/l) |
|---|---|---|
| Serum | 142 | 4.5 |
| Normal saline | 154 | 0 |
| Dextrose saline | 30 | 0 |
| 5% dextrose | 0 | 0 |
| Hartmann's | 130 | 5 |
| Gelofusine | 154 | 0 |

# HYPOVOLAEMIC SHOCK

**149** B – Class II hypovolaemic shock

**150** A – Class I hypovolaemic shock

**151** C – Class III hypovolaemic shock

The features of the different classes of hypovolaemic shock are shown in the table below.

**Table 2**

|  | Class I | Class II | Class III | Class IV |
|---|---|---|---|---|
| Pulse | <100 | >100 | >120 | >140 |
| Blood pressure | Normal | Normal | Decreased | Decreased |
| Pulse pressure | Normal | Decreased | Decreased | Decreased |
| Respiratory rate | 14-20 | 20-30 | 30-40 | >40 |

## NUTRITIONAL SUPPORT

**152**  C – Nasojejunal feeding

This condition will require medium-term feeding, and needs a method which infuses food distal to the pancreas.

**153**  E – PEG feeding

PEG feeding is the best option for long-term feeding.

**154**  A – Jejunostomy

Indications for jejunostomy include major upper abdominal surgery, major abdominal trauma, post-operative chemotherapy or radiotherapy and malnourished patients undergoing abdominal surgery.

**155**  F – TPN

There is no other appropriate route but TPN, as the small bowel is affected.

# THYROID NEOPLASMS

**156** F – Papillary carcinoma

Papillary carcinoma is characterised by Psammoma bodies. It is more common in women aged 20–50 years.

**157** A – Anaplastic carcinoma

Anaplastic carcinoma presents more commonly in the older patient and is aggressive, often presenting with dysphagia, dysphonia or stridor.

**158** D – Medullary carcinoma

The raised calcitonin level indicated medullary carcinoma.

# NIPPLE DISCHARGE

**159**   C – Intra-ductal papilloma

This is a benign neoplasm associated with bloody single-duct discharge.

**160**   D – Peri-ductal mastitis

Peri-ductal mastitis is strongly associated with smoking, and it causes a purulent discharge.

**161**   A – Ductal carcinoma in situ

A bloody discharge should be assumed to be from a malignancy until proved otherwise.

**162**   F – Prolactinoma

Essential lactation unrelated to childbirth and that the patient has systemic symptoms are consistent with the cause of the discharge being part of an endocrine process.

## SHOULDER PAIN

**163** A – Acute calcific tendonitis

This condition arises without injury, and is acutely very painful. It is more common in women and those in their third or fourth decades.

**164** B – Acute dislocation

The player has sustained a direct blow causing an acute dislocation, which is characterised by flattening of the normal shape of the deltoid.

**165** C – Frozen shoulder

Frozen shoulder often presents following minor trauma in elderly people. The pain is often worse at night, and abduction and external rotation are the movements worst affected.

# ASA GRADING – CLASSIFICATION OF PHYSICAL STATUS

*ASA grading is used by anaesthetists to place patients in certain groups according to their pre-operative physical condition, irrespective of the type of surgery they are planned to undergo.*

*Class 1 – normal, healthy individual.*

*Class 2 – patient with mild systemic disease.*

*Class 3 – patient with severe systemic disease that limits activity but is not incapacitating.*

*Class 4 – patient with incapacitating disease that is a constant threat to life.*

*Class 5 – moribund patient who is not expected to survive without an operation.*

**166**   D – Class 4

**167**   B – Class 2

**168**   A – Class 1

**169**   B – Class 2

**170**   C – Class 3

# STAGING OF TRANSITIONAL CELL CARCINOMA OF BLADDER

*Staging of bladder cancer depends on how far into the bladder wall the tumour has invaded. During TURBT the tumours should be carefully resected in layers to get specimens for accurate staging and to fully remove the more superficial tumours. Staging is as follows:*

$T_{is}$ – *in situ*

$T_a$ – *confined to epithelium*

$T_1$ – *invading lamina propria*

$T_{2a}$ – *invading superficial muscle*

$T_{2b}$ – *invading deep muscle*

$T_{3a}$ – *microscopic perivesical invasion*

$T_{3b}$ – *macroscopic perivesical invasion*

$T_{4a}$ – *invasion into adjacent organs*

$T_{4b}$ – *fixed to pelvic side wall.*

**171** H – $T_{4b}$

**172** C – $T_{2a}$

# PANCREATIC TUMOURS

**173**   G – Zollinger-Ellison tumour

**174**   E – Insulinoma

**175**   D – Glucagonoma

Pancreatic tumours may be benign or malignant. Benign tumours include adenomas, cystadenomas, insulinomas, glucagonomas and VIP-omas. Malignant tumours may be primary or secondary. Insulinomas are tumours of the B-cells of the pancreas and are usually solitary. They present with symptoms of hypoglycaemia including disturbed conciousness and odd behaviour, yet are completely normal between attacks. Gastrinomas are tumours of the non B-cells of the pancreatic islets and result in excess gastrin production. They usually present with peptic ulceration but also as diarrhoea, GI bleeds and perforation. They tend to have multiple metastases. Glucagonomas are tumours of the pancreatic alpha cells. They are very rare and present with an eczematous rash, glossitis, stomatitis and diabetes. They should be treated surgically due to their malignant potential.

# POLYPS

**176**   D – Juvenile polyp

**177**   A – Fibroma

**178**   B – Hyperplastic polyp

A polyp is defined as an abnormal elevation from an epithelial surface and can be malignant or benign. Hyperplastic polyps are the most common type. They are flat and the same colour as the bowel mucosa. They do not undergo malignant change. Juvenile polyps are typically found in children under ten years. They are usually present in the rectum but may be found anywhere in the large bowel, They are also not pre-malignant. Fibromas are rare colonic tumours arising from the submucosal layer. They are hard, mobile and pedunculated and rarely undergo malignant change. Peutz-Jegher's polyps are associated with the familial disorder and are associated with buccal hyperpigmentation. The polyps are most commonly found in the small bowel and are usually multiple. They have a low grade malignant potential.

# RADIOLOGICAL APPEARANCES

**179**   F – Sigmoid volvulus

**180**   G – Ulcerative colitis

Sigmoid volvulus is identified as a loop of distended bowel and the 'beak sign' on instant enema. Features indicating ulcerative colitis are loss of haustral fold pattern, mucosal irregularity, tubular ('lead pipe') shaped colon and no faecal residue within affected segment of bowel. Intramural gas is a sign of necrotising enterocolitis which affects neonates. Hirschsprung disease can be diagnosed by the presence of of a 'cone' between the collapsed distal and dilated proximal bowel on contrast enema – due to the portion of aganglionic bowel. Duodenal atresia is also seen in newborns and is picked up by the presence of a 'double bubble' on abdominal X-ray which consists of and air filled stomach and first part of the duodenum. Diverticular disease cannot be diagnosed on plain AXR but often appears as segmental lumen narrowing and tethered mucosa on gastrograffin enema.

# ANSWERS
# PRACTICE PAPER 3

## URINARY TRACT INFECTIONS

**1**     E – *Proteus* spp.

Staghorn calculi occur in strongly alkaline urine. They are usually associated with bacteria that produce urease, which breaks down urea to form ammonia. *Proteus* is the most common of these.

**2**     D – *Mycobacterium tuberculosis*

HIV patients and other immunocompromised patients are particularly susceptible to tuberculosis. Tuberculosis should always be suspected in patients with sterile pyuria in the absence of any other demonstrable abnormality.

**3**     F – *Schistosoma haematobium*

Schistosomiasis is endemic to the Middle East, Egypt in particular. The parasite lays eggs in the urinary tract, causing irritation. It may lead to squamous metaplasia, stone disease, or, if left untreated, squamous cell carcinoma.

# ANTIBIOTIC USE

**4**    A – 7-day course of antibiotics

Open fractures are contaminated wounds, therefore infection is assumed and treated. Besides surgical wound toilet, a course of antibiotics is required.

**5**    C – No prophylaxis required

An elective hernia repair is a clean procedure. A fresh incision is made to the skin, and bowel contents are kept within the bowel. If no mesh is used, as is the case in most femoral hernia repairs, there is no need for prophylactic antibiotics.

**6**    C – No prophylaxis required

There is no evidence that antibiotic prophylaxis prevents meningitis following fractures of the base of skull. There is, however, evidence that when prophylaxis is used, meningitis is caused by resistant strains of bacteria. Hence, antibiotic prophylaxis should not be used.

**7**    B – Antibiotics for 24 hours

This operation consists of implantation of a prosthetic graft. Infections in prosthetic grafts can be devastating, hence it is usual to give 24 hours of antibiotics; these are mostly first- or second-generation cephalosporins. Longer prophylaxis is unnecessary.

# DYSPHAGIA

**8**    F – Oesophageal carcinoma

Oesophageal carcinoma is commoner in smokers, those with increased alcohol intake, oesophageal strictures and some dietary deficiencies. Symptoms include dysphagia, retrosternal discomfort, chest pain, aspiration pneumonia and recurrent laryngeal nerve palsy. Prognosis is poor as the tumour readily metastasises.

**9**    G – Pharyngeal pouch

A pharyngeal pouch occurs in a weakness in the inferior constrictor muscle. It is also known as 'Killian's dehiscence'. It is commoner in males and usual features are halitosis (secondary to the retention of undigested food in the oesophagus), recurrent sore throats, regurgitation of undigested food (sometimes eaten days before), aspiration pneumonia and neck swelling. Treatment is by excision of the pouch.

**10**    A – Achalasia

Achalasia is a dysmotility disorder of the lower oesophagus. It is of unknown pathogenesis but predisposes to carcinomatous change. Barium swallow shows the typical bird's beak appearance, while manometry shows abnormally high intra-oesophageal resting pressure. Treatment is by balloon dilatation, Heller's cardiomyotomy or, more recently, injection of botulinum toxin.

# INCONTINENCE

## 11    B – Bladder outlet obstruction

This man has typical symptoms of an enlarged prostate – reduced flow, increased frequency and incomplete emptying. The most likely explanation is bladder outlet obstruction caused by the enlarge prostate with overflow incontinence.

## 12    D – Neurogenic incontinence

Multiple sclerosis is a common cause of a neuropathic bladder. The absence of voiding urge supports this diagnosis.

## 13    F – Small bladder capacity

Interstitial cystitis reduces the compliance of the bladder leading to a smaller bladder capacity. This leads to high filling pressures for the same volume of urine.

## 14    C – Genuine stress incontinence

Genuine stress incontinence is usually due to lax pelvic floor muscles. This is especially common in multi-parous women who have had multiple vaginal deliveries.

## 15    B – Bladder outlet obstruction

The poor flow and high residual volume of urine indicate bladder outlet obstruction. Gonorrhoea can cause urethral strictures leading to bladder outlet obstruction in severe cases.

# PRE-OPERATIVE INVESTIGATIONS

**16**    A – ECG

An ECG is required for anyone over the age of 50 likely to have a general anaesthetic. The procedure itself is relatively minor and not likely to involve any major body fluid losses. As the man is otherwise healthy, no other investigations are necessary.

**17**    G – No investigation required

This patient is a fit and healthy individual under the age of 40. No investigations are required. The chest infection is transient and does not require further investigation, although it would be appropriate to delay surgery until he has fully recovered from his infection.

**18**    C – ECG + FBC + U&E

ECG + FBC + U&E are the minimum required investigations for anyone undergoing major surgery. Other investigations such as chest X-ray, spirometry and urinalysis should also be considered.

# TREATMENT OF ULCERS

## 19    E – Total contact casting

This foot ulcer in a diabetic patient with peripheral neuropathy is likely to be due to a combination of microvascular disease and the neuropathy. Treatment of this type of ulcer is usually based on off-loading the affected area, hence the use of a total contact cast. In addition tight diabetic control would be helpful.

## 20    D – Revascularisation

Although this ulcer has many characteristics of a venous ulcer, the ABPI is low. This indicates an arterial element to the ulcer. Compression bandaging in this case would further compromise the circulation. Revascularisation is needed and if successful, compression bandaging may be undertaken afterwards.

## 21    A – Compression bandaging

This is a venous type ulcer. The duplex shows good arterial flow, hence compression bandaging would be suitable treatment.

## 22    C – Excision

This history is compatible with malignant change in a chronic ulcer. Surgical excision would be the most appropriate, and skin grafting may be required afterwards.

## 23    D – Revascularisation

This is an arterial ulcer with stigmata of chronic arterial insufficiency. Revascularisation should be attempted, either endovascularly or surgically.

# SURGICALLY IMPORTANT ORGANISMS

**24**    A – *Acinetobacter*

*Acinetobacter* is an environmental micro-organism that is resistant to many antibiotics. It often is the cause of outbreaks of multidrug-resistant infection in ICUs. Systemic invasion is common.

**25**    H – *Staphylococcus epidermidis*

*Staphylococcus epidermidis* is a commensal of the skin and is normally non-virulent. It is often responsible for infections involving prostheses, either joints or grafts. *Staphylococcus aureus* is coagulase positive.

**26**    B – *Bacteroides fragilis*

*Bacteroides fragilis* is the commonest organism causing serious anaerobic infection. It is particularly common after abdominal or gynaecological procedures. It produces $\beta$-lactamase and is therefore penicillin resistant.

**27**    D – Fusobacteria

Tonsillar infection is called Vincent's angina. *Fusobacterium fusiformis* and *Borrelia vincentii* are the two usual causes. *Fusobacterium fusiformis* is a Gram-negative rod-shaped organism.

**28**    F – *Pseudomonas aeruginosa*

*Pseudomonas aeruginosa* is a Gram-negative bacillus, and is a commensal to human and animal gastrointestinal tracts, water and the soil. It is a common pathogen in immunocompromised patients and those with other underlying pathology. It is resistant to most antibiotics.

## CORD LESIONS

### 29    B – Brown–Séquard syndrome

In this scenario there is hemisection of the cord, resulting in paralysis on the affected side below the lesion, along with loss of proprioception and fine discrimination. Pain and temperature sensation are lost on the opposite side as the spinothalamic tract carries fibres which have decussated at a lower level.

### 30    E – Posterior cord syndrome

Hyperextension injuries with fractures of the posterior vertebral elements commonly cause posterior cord syndrome. The posterior columns are affected, hence proprioception is affected causing the profound ataxia.

### 31    A – Anterior cord syndrome

Anterior cord syndrome is common after compression fractures of the vertebral bodies. There is often damage to the anterior spinal artery, hence the neurological damage is a combination of direct trauma and ischaemic damage. Corticospinal and spinothalamic tracts are involved causing loss of power and reduction in pain and temperature sensation below the affected level.

### 32    D – Central cord syndrome

Central cord syndrome is usually seen in older patients with cervical spondylosis. The cord may be compressed by an osteophyte and intervertebral disc anteriorly and ligamentum flavum posteriorly. This results in flaccid weakness of the arms but preservation of motor and sensory fibres to the lower limb, as these are located more peripherally in the cord.

# WOUND COVERAGE

**33** D – Rectus abdominis flap

A myocutaneous flap is the method of choice for simultaneous breast reconstruction. Given that she is a keen sportswoman, and especially a climber, the latissimus dorsi flap would cause significant impairment, as this is one of the main climbing muscles. A rectus abdominis flap would therefore be preferred.

**34** E – Split-skin graft

A split-skin graft is the easiest method of wound coverage in this case. As there is healthy muscle under the wound, a split-skin graft should take.

# BENIGN ANO-RECTAL CONDITIONS

## 35    A – DeLorme's procedure

DeLorme's procedure involves excising the excess prolapsed rectal mucosa, with the underlying muscle being sutured up in a concertina fashion.

## 36    B – Diltiazem ointment

Fissure-in-ano is a common condition. Pain on defaecation is the most common symptom, and others include pruritus ani, minor bleeding and constipation secondary to pain. It is the most common lesion in Crohn's disease. Treatment is usually medical: either diltiazem cream or glycerol trinitrate ointment. In addition, stool-bulking agents may be used to ease the constipation.

## 37    F – Rubber band ligation

This is a classic history of haemorrhoids. They are normally found at the 3, 7 and 11 o'clock positions in the anal canal. First-line treatment usually consists of rubber band ligation or injection with sclerosants. Persistent, troublesome haemorrhoids may be treated with haemorrhoidectomy.

## 38    D – Incision and drainage

Inter-sphincteric abscesses can be incised, drained and laid open. Trans-sphincteric abscesses are usually laid open to reduce the risk of incontinence following damage to both internal and external sphincter mechanisms. In this case seton drainage is used, where a suture is tied along the line of the fistula.

# TYPES OF CHEST TRAUMA

## 39    H – Tension pneumothorax

This man has a flail chest. The positive intrathoracic pressure produced by intubation and artificial ventilation is likely to have caused a tension pneumothorax. Intubation in this kind of scenario is usually covered by insertion of a chest drain.

## 40    B – Cardiac tamponade

This is a classic picture of cardiac tamponade. Blood collects in the pericardium, causing muffled heart sounds, increased CVP and decreased systolic blood pressure. Aspiration of as little as 15 ml of blood can produce significant symptomatic relief.

## 41    I – Tracheobronchial tree injury

The chest drain is in the correct position. Despite this, there is evidence of a large air leak given the increasing size of the pneumothorax. Tracheobronchial injury is likely. This may require insertion of more than one chest drain until definitive treatment can be achieved.

# PAIN IN THE RIGHT UPPER QUADRANT

## 42    C – Biliary colic

Biliary colic causes RUQ pain without pyrexia, jaundice is not uncommon if the calculus obstructs the common bile duct.

## 43    B – Ascending cholangitis

RUQ pain associated with jaundice points to a biliary cause, but the lack of a calculus in the  common bile duct rules out cholecystitis.

## 44    J – Subphrenic abscess

Subphrenic abscess is a known complication of diverticular disease, usually occurring approximately 1–3 weeks following the initial episode.

## 45    A – Acute pancreatitis

Amylase of >1000 somorgyi u d/L is characteristic of acute pancreatitis.

## 46    G – Lower lobe pneumonia

The fact the patient has no rigors, and no other signs of disease in the RUQ, suggest an infective cause which can refer pain to the RUQ.

# SKIN INCISIONS

**47**     I – Upper midline incision

The diagnosis is likely to be a perforated peptic ulcer secondary to NSAID use. This woman requires an oversew of the ulcer. The best exposure to perform this would be via an upper midline laparotomy, which could be extended if required.

**48**     E – Kocher's incision

Kocher's incision is a right subcostal incision. There are usually three more portals placed for laparoscopic surgery besides the peri-umbilical one. These are usually approximately 3 cm below the right sub-costal margin. These portal incisions can be joined together for an incision roughly akin to Kocher's.

**49**     C – Lower midline incision

The likely diagnosis is either a stercoral perforation or a malignant perforation. Both are likely to involve the sigmoid colon, and this is best exposed using a lower midline incision. Again, this can be extended if required.

**50**     A – Lanz's incision

This is a classic history of acute appendicitis. Lanz's incision is possibly the best incision cosmetically for removing the appendix. It is a slightly oblique incision centred just below McBurney's point two-thirds of the way from the umbilicus to the anterior superior iliac spine.

# VENTILATORS

### 51    A – ASB

ASB is a pressure-controlled, flow-cycled mode of ventilation. The patient is required to breathe for themselves in this method. It can be combined with either BIPAP or SIMV to support spontaneous breaths that occur during these modes of ventilation.

### 52    C – CMV

This is generally reserved for use in operating theatres alone, as it is difficult to wean patients using this method of ventilation only. It operates on either a set volume or a set inspiratory pressure. There is no active patient interaction.

### 53    D – CPAP

CPAP is one of the simplest forms of ventilation. It uses a facemask and provides a continuous positive pressure. It improves the compliance of the lungs, thereby reducing the work of breathing. It can also help with opening up collapsed alveoli in cases of atelectasis.

### 54    G – SIMV

SIMV requires the tidal volume and rate to be set, but there is also a time set between each breath during which, if the patient initiates a spontaneous breath the mandatory breath is synchronised with this. This allows for patient–machine inter-activity and the patient can be effectively weaned by increasing the time between each mandatory breath.

# SALIVARY GLAND SWELLINGS

**55**    D – Frey's syndrome

Frey's syndrome or gustatory sweating may occur after surgery to the parotid gland. Flushing and sweating usually occur along the distribution of the auriculo-temporal nerve. Damage to this nerve has been postulated to be a cause.

**56**    C – Acute viral sialadenitis

Acute viral sialadenitis, better known as mumps, causes orchitis in 20% of post-pubertal men. Mumps can be distinguished from other forms of acute parotitis by the absence of a neutrophil leucocytosis.

**57**    H – Sjögren's syndrome

Secondary Sjögren's syndrome is associated with connective tissue disorders such as SLE and rheumatoid arthritis. Its features consist of dry eyes and a dry mouth.

**58**    E – Mikulicz's syndrome

Mikulicz's disease is a triad consisting of symmetrical enlargement of all salivary glands, narrowing of the palpebral fissures secondary to lacrimal gland enlargement and parchment-like dryness of the mouth. In Mikulicz's syndrome there is enlargement of the glands secondary to leukaemia or generalised disease. Mikulicz's disease is due to an autoimmune process in the salivary glands.

**59**    G – Sialolithiasis

Stone formation in the salivary glands usually occurs in the submandibular gland, but can occur in any. Just before meals, salivation is stimulated, causing saliva to build up behind the obstruction resulting in swelling and increased pain.

# MANAGEMENT OF CHEST TRAUMA

**60**    G – Needle thoracocentesis

This man has signs of a tension pneumothorax. Hyper-resonance, absence of breath sounds and tracheal deviation all support the diagnosis. He has already had a needle thoracocentesis, but during transfer the cannula may have displaced or occluded. A further attempt at needle thoracocentesis should be made. Definitive treatment is with a chest drain.

**61**    I – Urgent arteriography

This man may have traumatic aortic rupture. The widened mediastinum, left haemothorax and deviation of the trachea to the right support this diagnosis. Although this patient appears stable, it is imperative that further assessment of his aorta is carried out by means of either a CT scan or arteriography. Patients with aortic injury who have a chance of survival usually have an incomplete laceration near the ligamentum arteriosum of the aorta. Specific signs are frequently absent and further investigation is warranted if aortic injury is suspected.

**62**    D – Immediate open thoracotomy

Patients with penetrating thoracic injuries who present with cardiac arrest or pulseless electrical activity are candidates for immediate open thoracotomy. Closed cardio-pulmonary resuscitation would not be effective in this situation. A left anterior thoracotomy is the procedure of choice with ongoing resuscitation procedures.

# CARCINOGENS

## 63    C – Carcinoma of the bladder

Schistosomes are parasites which invade the urinary tract, and can lay eggs in the bladder. Schistosomiasis is associated with chronic inflammation of the bladder and squamous cell carcinoma of the bladder.

## 64    C – Carcinoma of the bladder

B-naphthylamine is converted to the active carcinogen 1-hydroxy–2-naphthylamine in the liver, but glucuronidation of the compound in the liver offers some protection. In the bladder, glucuronidase unconjugates the molecule, and the active carcinogen is concentrated, exposing the urothelium of the bladder to carcinogenic effects.

## 65    B – Burkitt's lymphoma

Epstein–Barr virus is associated with Burkitt's lymphoma in the presence of malarial infection.

## 66    E – MALT tumour

There is a link between *Helicobacter pylori* infection and gastric carcinoma, but it has a stronger association with the so-called MALT lymphoma. It has been shown that MALT lymphomas sometimes regress with *Helicobacter pylori* infection treatment.

## 67    F – Hepatocellular carcinoma

*Aspergillus flavus* releases aflatoxin, which occur as dietary contaminants and are associated with hepatocellular carcinoma.

## 68    H – Oropharyngeal carcinoma

Betel nuts are chewed in parts of Asia as an alternative to tobacco. This is associated with a higher incidence of oropharyngeal carcinoma.

# INOTROPES

**69** A – Adrenaline

Adrenaline has strong $\beta$-adrenergic effects and is mainly used as a bronchodilator in anaphylactic shock.

**70** A – Adrenaline

Adrenaline has a propensity to cause arrhythmia. It is for this reason that adrenaline is used in cardiac arrest situations to try to convert a non-shockable rhythm to ventricular fibrillation – which is susceptible to electrical shock.

**71** C – Dopamine

Stimulation of dopaminergic receptors leads to increased renal blood flow, hence increased glomerular filtration rate and increased sodium excretion. However, at higher doses, $\beta_1$-receptors are also stimulated, causing an increase in heart rate and contractility, and at very high doses (>10 $\mu$g/kg per min) dopamine stimulates $\alpha_1$-receptors causing reduced tissue perfusion and therefore reducing glomerular filtration rate.

**72** E – Noradrenaline

Noradrenaline is a powerful $\alpha_1$ stimulant, and causes strong vasoconstriction. It causes increases in both systolic and diastolic pressure, but also reduces renal blood flow. It is mainly used in the treatment of shock.

# SCROTAL SWELLINGS

### 73 E – Testicular torsion

Testicular torsion usually presents as an exquisitely tender testis which may be lying horizontally or high-riding. There may be a history of trauma.

### 74 C – Hydrocoele

Primary hydrocoeles are most common over the age of 40. The swelling fills one side of the scrotum. Fluid collects in the tunica vaginalis hence giving a fluctuant swelling which transilluminates.

### 75 B – Fournier's gangrene

Fournier's gangrene is necrotising fasciitis of the scrotum. It is caused by a mixed infection in the deep fascia and skin of the perineum, scrotum and penis. Patients may present in septic shock.

# TRAUMA

## 76 E – Intubation

This man has a GCS of 3. He is unable to protect his own airway; hence securing the airway is paramount.

## 77 C – Full spinal and neurological assessment

Calcaneal fractures are high energy injuries. They are associated with injuries throughout the spinal column; hence a full spinal/neurological assessment should be carried out.

## 78 B – CT scan of the head

This man has a GCS of 11 (eye opening 2, verbal 4, best motor 5). The sudden drop in GCS may indicate an intra-cranial haemorrhage. A lucid interval such as this is common with extra-dural haemorrhage and a CT scan is indicated.

# LOCAL ANAESTHETICS

**79**   B – 10 ml

The maximum recommended dose of lidocaine as given in the *British National Formulary* is 200 mg. This equates to 10 ml of 2% lidocaine.

**80**   D – 30 ml

The maximum recommended dose of bupivacaine as given in the *British National Formulary* is 150 mg. This is equivalent to 30 ml of 0.5% bupivacaine.

**81**   H – 80 ml

With the addition of adrenaline, the maximum safe dose increases to 200 mg. This equates to 80 ml of 0.25% bupivacaine solution.

**82**   F – 50 ml

With the addition of adrenaline, the maximum safe dose of lidocaine is 500 mg. This equates to 50 ml of 1% lidocaine solution.

## PERIPHERAL NERVE INJURY

### 83    A – Axillary nerve

The axillary nerve may be damaged in up to 5% of dislocations of the shoulder, and damage to the nerve produces sensory loss in the 'regimental patch' area. This is on the lateral aspect of the arm around the lower border of the deltoid muscle.

### 84    D – Posterior interosseous nerve of the forearm

The posterior interosseous nerve passes around the neck of the radius and is susceptible to injury here. It supplies most of the extensors of the wrist and fingers, although the extensor carpi radialis longus is supplied by the radial nerve before it divides, hence some wrist extension remains. The posterior interosseous nerve is purely motor, therefore no sensation is lost.

### 85    A – Axillary nerve

The axillary nerve wraps around the surgical neck of the humerus and is susceptible to injury here. It supplies the deltoid muscle, hence damage to this nerve limits abduction.

### 86    F – Ulnar nerve

The ulnar nerve runs just behind the medial epicondyle. Damage to the nerve produces a typical 'claw' hand, with unopposed action of the extensors and paralysis of the deep flexors to the ring and little fingers in conjunction with paralysis of the lumbricals and interossei.

### 87    B – Median nerve

The median nerve crosses the brachial artery anteriorly in the arm. Hence pulsatile bleeding suggesting brachial artery damage is likely to damage the median nerve.

# CHEMOTHERAPY

### 88   C – No chemotherapy

Chemotherapy is usually offered in invasive carcinoma of the breast with lymph node involvement.

### 89   A – Adjuvant chemotherapy

Currently chemotherapy is offered for all Duke's C carcinomas and Duke's B carcinomas with poor prognostic indicators. These include perforation, vascular invasion and poor differentiation.

### 90   C – No chemotherapy

Chemotherapy would not be offered in this case as the micrometastases were not detected on routine scanning. Therefore, it would not be possible to monitor response to treatment.

# DIAGNOSIS OF ENDOCRINE DISORDERS

**91**    A – 24-hour VMA

Phaeochromocytomas are tumours of the adrenal medulla arising from chromaffin cells and secrete excess catecholamines. VMA is a breakdown product of catecholamines and therefore urinary levels become elevated.

**92**    F – Short Synacthen test

Addison's disease is often associated with other autoimmune disorders. It can be investigated for by using the short Synacthen test which does not cause a rise in plasma cortisol in affected patients whereas it does in unaffected people.

**93**    C – Plasma aldosterone levels

Diagnosis of Conn's syndrome (aldosterone-secreting adrenocortical adenoma) is made by measuring plasma aldosterone, and CT or MRI to localise the adenoma.

**94**    D – Radio-immunoassay of 17-hydroxyprogesterone

Congenital adrenal hyperplasia occurs as a result of 2,1-hydroxylase deficiency. 17-Hydroxyprogesterone levels are found to be elevated.

**95**    B – Dexamethasone suppression test

This is a typical presentation of someone with Cushing's syndrome. Cushing's syndrome can be diagnosed either by measuring 24-hour urinary free cortisol or by an overnight dexamethasone suppression test which fails to suppress morning cortisol levels in affected patients.

# TERMS USED FOR DISORDERS OF GROWTH AND DIFFERENTIATION

**96**   D – Hyperplasia

Hyperplasia is increased tissue or organ size due to increased cell divisions, in response to increased functional demand. This is different from hypertrophy, which is an increase in cell size without replication.

**97**   B – Atrophy

Atophy is the decrease in size of an organ or tissue by reduction in cell size and/or reduction in cell numbers. It often involves apoptosis and occurs in both pathological and physiological conditions.

**98**   G – Metaplasia

Metaplasia is the reversible transformation of one type of terminally differentiated cell type. It often occurs in response to environmental stress.

**99**   A – Agenesis

Agenesis is the failure of development of an organ or structure. This differs from atresia which is failure of development of a lumen in a normally tubular structure.

# TREATMENT OF ANAL CONDITIONS

### 100   B – GTN ointment

Anal fissures are generally found in the midline posteriorly, but anterior fissures are seen in women. First-line treatment is GTN ointment, which reduces spasm of the anal muscles allowing the damaged mucosa to receive a good blood supply which it needs to heal. Efforts should be made to keep stools soft and prevent constipation. Dilatation of the anus under general anaesthetic or lateral sphincterotomy can also be done but since both can result in incontinence they are best considered a last resort particularly in women.

### 101   G – Seton insertion

History of multiple perianal abscesses and then persistent purulent discharge is highly suggestive of a fistula-in-ano. MRI is the best means of assessing the fistula tracts which enables management to be planned. Fistulae running above puborectalis (supra-sphincteric and high trans-sphincteric fistulae) cannot be treated by laying them open as the internal sphincter will be disrupted leading to incontinence. Instead they can be treated with seton insertion, which drains the infection and allows healing. This is then removed several weeks later leaving a simple track which should then heal.

## LOWER LIMB NEUROPATHY

### 102   A – Common peroneal nerve

The common peroneal nerve is in danger of compression when applying below-knee casts. It is vulnerable around the neck of the fibula. Both branches of the peroneal nerve are therefore affected, compromising dorsiflexion (deep peroneal nerve) and eversion (superficial peroneal nerve).

### 103   F – Sural nerve

The sural nerve is a cutaneous sensory branch of the tibial nerve. It runs just posterior to the short saphenous vein in the leg, hence is vulnerable to damage during avulsion of this vein.

### 104   D – Sciatic nerve

The sciatic nerve is particularly vulnerable in fracture dislocations of the hip. Damage to the nerve has been reported in up to 16% of cases. The quadriceps are spared as they are supplied by the femoral nerve, and its cutaneous branch, the saphenous nerve, supplies sensation to the upper calf and medial aspect of the leg.

### 105   C – Saphenous nerve

The long saphenous vein is the most commonly used vein for vein grafting procedures. The saphenous nerve runs in close proximity to the vein, supplying the upper calf and medial aspect of the leg. It is vulnerable to damage when the vein is stripped, particularly if it is stripped below the knee.

# MANAGEMENT OF FRACTURED NECK OF FEMUR

*The way in which a fractured neck of femur is managed is dictated by the blood supply to the femoral head. A significant amount of the blood supply comes from the retinacular vessels which pass proximally within the joint capsule. These vessels are therefore disrupted in intra-capsular (subcapital) fractures.*

## 106    E – Open reduction and internal fixation

Undisplaced subcapital fractures have a good chance of maintaining the blood supply as there is minimal disruption of the capsule. They can generally be treated with insertion of cannulated screws. In a displaced fracture (ie Garden's III and IV) there is a high risk of developing avascular necrosis of the femoral head and so hemiarthroplasty is the preferred management. The exception to this is in young patients for whom preservation of their own femoral head rather than insertion of a prosthesis at a young age is a better option. In such circumstances the fracture may require open reduction before internal fixation, for example with cannulated screws.

## 107    D – Hemiarthroplasty

See answer 106 for explanation.

## 108    C – Dynamic hip screw

Inter-trochanteric (extracapsular) fractures are fixed with a dynamic hip screw after closed reduction on a fracture table.

## 109    E – Open reduction and internal fixation

Subtrochanteric extension of a fracture renders it highly unstable therefore unsuitable for dynamic hip screw. It requires open reduction and internal fixation, eg with an intermedullary hip screw.

# CONDITIONS CAUSED BY MICROBES

**110**   A – *Candida albicans*

Oral candidiasis (thrush) is seen in neonates and immunocompromised patients, or those on long-term antibiotics. It presents as white plaques on the mucous membrane.

**111**   H – *Streptococcus pyogenes*

Wound infection and surrounding inflammation (cellulitis) is commonly caused by *Streptococcus pyogenes*. This bacteria also causes tonsillitis, otitis media, erysipelas and necrotising fasciitis.

**112**   D – *Escherichia coli*

*E. coli* is the causative organism in 90% of community acquired urinary tract infections and 50 % of hospital acquired infections. Female diabetics are three times more likely to have a UTI than non-diabetics.

**113**   C – *Clostridium perfringens*

*Clostridium perfringens* is a normal bowel inhabitant. However, when present in an anaerobic environment such as a wound, its spores get converted into toxin-producing pathogens. The toxins destroy the surrounding microcirculation. Gas formation occurs with local crepitus.

**114**   B – *Clostridium difficile*

*Clostridium difficile* causes a diarrhoea which is generally associated with broad spectrum antibiotic use. The best method of diagnosis is the demonstration of specific clostridium difficile toxin in the faeces.

**115**   E – *Helicobacter pylori*

*Helicobacter pylori* is a gram negative, spirally shaped bacterium which colonises the gastric mucosa. It can cause gastritis, duodenal ulceration and puts patients at risk of developing gastric ulcers and carcinoma.

# HYPERSENSITIVITY REACTIONS

**116**    D – Type IV hypersensitivity reaction

This type of reaction is also called 'cell mediated' and is mediated by T-cells which have been previously sensitised by an allergen. They activate cytotoxic T-cells which recruit and activate macrophages.

**117**    C – Type III hypersensitivity reaction

This type of reaction is also called 'immune complex mediated'. It results in the formation of antigen-antibody complexes in the circulation or at extravascular sites which leads to complement activation then neutrophil activation.

**118**    A – Type I hypersensitivity reaction

Type I reactions are also known as 'immediate' reactions. The body forms IgE in response to exposu to a certain allergen. IgE then binds to mast cells and basophils so that when there is re-exposure to the allergens, inflammatory mediators are released from the basophils and mast cells.

**119**    D – Type IV hypersensitivity reaction

See answer to Q 116

**120**    A – Type I hypersensitivity reaction

See answer to Q 118

**121**    B – Type II hypersensitivity reaction

Type 11 reactions are also known as 'cytotoxic' reactions. They are mediated by antibodies formed against antigens. Tissue damage then results via a variety of mechanisms including complement and antibody-dependent cell-mediated cytotoxicity.

# MANAGEMENT OF VASCULAR DISEASE

**122** B – Medical management (diabetic and blood pressure control, aspirin, statin) and regular follow-up

Elective surgery is normally carried out for AAA only if the patient is relatively fit and has an aneurysm greater than 5.5 cm in diameter as the mortality for the operation is 5%.

**123** D – Surgery after further investigation

Overall mortality in ruptured aneurysms is 75% and unstable patients should proceed to urgent surgery. Ultrasound scan or CT scan should be carried out if there is any doubt about the diagnosis and the patient is stable.

**124** B – Medical management (diabetic and blood pressure control, aspirin, statin) and regular follow-up

Recent trials have shown benefit of medical management but no benefit of surgical management in the treatment of patients with 10–70% carotid stenosis. Those who should be offered surgery are those with 70–99% stenosis who have recently become symptomatic.

**125** D – Surgery after further investigation

As duplex scanning is highly operator dependent, those who are borderline on duplex scan should undergo an additional form of investigation.

## GLASGOW COMA SCALE SCORES

The Glasgow Coma Scale (GCS) is a system used to record and monitor a patient's level of consciousness. There are a total of 15 points based on four categories: best motor response (6 = obeys commands; 5 = localises to pain; 4 = withdraws from pain; 3 = abnormal flexion; 2 = abnormal extension; 1 = none), best verbal response (5 = orientated; 4 = confused; 3 = inappropriate speech; 2 = incomprehensible sounds; 1 = none) and best eye opening response (4 = open spontaneously; 3 = opens to speech; 2 = opens to painful stimulus; 1 = none). A GCS of 8 is an important score as it is at this point that you consider a patient for intubation as they are unlikely to be able to protect their own airway.

**126**   E – 10

**127**   B – 7

**128**   B – 7

**129**   F – 13

# MANAGEMENT OF TRANSITIONAL CELL CARCINOMA OF THE BLADDER

## 130   G – Nephro-urethrectomy

Transitional cell carcinomas of the renal pelvis resemble those affecting the bladder but are much less common. They tend to invade the renal parenchyma and have a tendency to distal spread. There is also a strong tendency for these tumours to be multifocal. Conventional surgical treatment is by nephro-ureterectomy and the ureter must be removed with a cuff of bladder wall.

## 131   C – Cystectomy + urethrectomy + ileal conduit

In patients who have primary CIS which is unresponsive to medical management cystectomy is an option. Often this is accompanied by urethrectomy as this is often also involved. Urine is commonly diverted into an ileal conduit.

## HAEMORRHAGIC SHOCK

**132**   C – Class III haemorrhagic shock

**133**   B – Class II haemorrhagic shock

**134**   C – Class III haemorrhagic shock

Reduction of blood volume is associated with physiological responses mainly mediated by the sympathetic nervous system, which aim to maintain blood pressure and hence blood supply to the vital organs. Haemorrhagic shock can be divided into four classes depending on the amount of blood lost. Each class is associated with particular parameters which help in the estimation of blood loss.

- Class I is loss of 0–15% of circulating volume and there are no obvious changes apart from the patient perhaps feeling uncomfortable and restless.

- Class II (15–30% loss) is associated with a rise in pulse rate to greater than 100 beats/min, urine output reduced to 20–30 ml/h and a raised respiratory rate of 20–30 breaths/min. The blood pressure is normal but pulse pressure is reduced.

- Class III (30–40% loss) is associated with a tachycardia of >120 beats/min, reduction in both pulse pressure and blood pressure and reduction in urine output to 10–20 ml/h.

- In Class IV (>40% blood loss) the patient becomes anxious and may be confused. There is tachycardia of >130 beats/min, blood pressure and pulse pressure are low and the patient is anuric. Respiratory rate is over 40 breaths/min.

# MANAGEMENT OF THYROID DISEASE

**135**   D – Propylthiouracil

First-line treatment for Graves' disease is carbimazole. In certain individuals it has the unfortunate side effect of agranulocytosis and so propylthiouracil is used instead.

**136**   D – Propylthiouracil

Propylthiouracil is also the drug of choice in pregnancy as it is protein bound and therefore less likely to cross the placenta.

**137**   E – Radio-iodide ablation

Radio-iodide ablation is safe for patients in whom medical management has failed and who are not planning on becoming pregnant during treatment.

**138**   F – Subtotal thyroidectomy

Surgery for thyroid disorders is carried out for cosmesis, compression symptoms, retrosternal extension and carcinoma.

# CAUSES OF JAUNDICE

**139  A – Carcinoma of head of the pancreas**

Painless jaundice together with a history of weight loss is strongly suggestive of a malignancy. Together with an obstructive picture (pale stools and dark urine) carcinoma of the head of the pancreas is the most likely diagnosis.

**140  B – Gallstones**

Jaundice in children with sickle cell disease may be due to red cell haemolysis. However, coupled with episodes of epigastric pain and an obstructive picture, the most likely diagnosis is gallstone obstruction of the common bile duct as pigment bile stones are common.

**141  F – Primary liver carcinoma**

Sharing of needles among intravenous drug misusers is a serious risk factor for hepatitis B and C, both of which predispose to the development of hepatocellular cancer in later years. $\alpha$-Fetoprotein is a marker for this cancer, although it is also raised in hepatoma.

# KNEE INJURIES

### 142   D – Medial meniscus tear

Tenderness over the joint line following an acute injury is most likely due to a meniscal injury rather than a collateral ligament. Bucket handle tears of menisci can result in positioning of the torn meniscus between the articular surfaces preventing full extension of the knee.

### 143   A – Anterior cruciate ligament tear

Anterior cruciate ligament tears result in rapid swelling of the affected knee. This is because the ligament is intra-articular and haemarthrosis can follow a tear. Hyper-extension is a classic mechanism by which these tears occur.

# TYPES OF ULCER

### 144　C – Marjolin's ulcer

Chronic ulcers are at risk of developing into a squamous cell carcinoma or Marjolin's ulcer. Changes such as raised, rolled edges with an increase in granulation tissue warrant further investigation.

### 145　B – Curling's ulcer

Severe burns predispose patients to developing 'stress' ulcers or Curling's ulcers.

### 146　A – Arterial ulcer

Diabetic patients are at risk of developing both neuropathic and arterial ulcers. Whereas neuropathic ulcers are painless, arterial ulcers are very painful, are located over pressure areas and have a classic 'punched-out' appearance.

# TREATMENT OF PROSTATE CANCER

## 147   E – Surveillance

Curative treatment for prostate cancer can only be offered to those with $T_1$ and $T_2$ disease (ie localised). Such patients can be managed by surveillance alone (DRE and regular PSA measurements) with further management when they become symptomatic or when PSA level rises. Radical prostatectomy is only usually offered to those with a life expectancy of > 10 years and is associated with a relatively high level of impotence and incontinence when compared with other treatments.

## 148   B – Brachytherapy

Localised disease can also be treated with radiotherapy in the form of external beam radiotherapy which requires the patient to attend hospital on a daily basis for 4–6 weeks or brachytherapy which involves the implantation of radioactive seeds into the prostate. For this treatment the prostate must be less than 50–60 grams as the pubic arch can prevent implantation. T3 and T4 (locally advanced and metastatic disease) can be treated with hormone manipulation using luteinising hormone releasing hormone agonist, anti-androgens or orchidectomy.

## 149   C – External beam radiotherapy

Radiotherapy can be used for symptomatic metastasis and hormone-relapsed cancer.

## MANAGEMENT OF ANKLE INJURIES

### 150   B – Closed reduction and plaster of paris

If an ankle fracture is stable (ie one malleolar affected or no talar shift), can be managed perfectly well by closed reduction and plaster cast.

### 151   C – Open reduction and internal fixation

Unstable fractures (ie those with talar shift, potential for talar shift or associated fibular fracture extending above the tibial plafond) require open reduction and internal fixation.

### 152   E – Support, NSAIDs and early mobilisation

Ankle sprains should be managed conservatively with analgesia with or without strapping and the patient should be encouraged to move the ankle and weight bear.

# HAEMORRHOIDS

**153**  D – Injection sclerotherapy

**154**  C – Haemorrhoidectomy

Haemorrhoids can be described as first, second or third degree (confined to anal canal, prolapse on defaecation, and reduce spontaneously or with digital reduction or permanently prolapsed, respectively). First-degree haemorrhoids can be treated with bulking agents and topical anaesthesia but if troublesome can be injected with oily phenol as an outpatient procedure. Second-degree haemorrhoids can be treated with rubber band ligation. Only approximately 5% of haemorrhoids require formal haemorrhoidectomy.

**155**  B – Evacuation of clot

Thrombosis of piles occurs when prolapsed piles become congested and oedematous and cannot be reduced. Venous return is obstructed and thrombosis occurs. This can be treated conservatively or by incision and evacuation of clot under local anaesthesia.

# COMPLICATIONS OF COLORECTAL CANCER

### 156   A – Appendicitis

Appendicitis is a complication of caecal carcinoma due to obstruction of the lumen. However, an important differential is perforation and formation of a localised abscess which can present with the same symptoms.

### 157   B – Colocolic intussusception

Intussusception typically presents as in this case and the tumour acts as the apex. Half (50%) of all adult intussusceptions are due to carcinoma.

### 158   C – Fistula formation

Direct invasion of a tumour into a neighbouring organ can cause a fistula, eg vesico-colic, rectovaginal or in the case in the question, fistulation of the transverse colon to the stomach or duodenum.

# ABNORMALITIES OF CALCIUM BALANCE

### 159   C – Hypoparathyroidism

Hypoparathyroidism presents with the symptoms of hypocalcaemia including paraesthesia, cramps, tetany, circumoral tingling and convulsions. Although most commonly seen post-operatively owing to damage to the parathyroid glands (eg post-thyroidectomy), hypoparathyroidism is also seen after acute pancreatitis, chronic renal failure and in vitamin D deficiency.

### 160   F – Tertiary hyperparathyroidism

Primary hyperparathyroidism is most commonly due to a single parathyroid adenoma causing raised levels of PTH and calcium. Secondary hyperparathyroidism is caused by chronic renal failure in response to a low calcium level and is characterised by a low serum calcium and a raised PTH level. Tertiary hyperparathyroidism is also seen in chronic renal failure and is due to the parathyroid gland becoming hyperplastic and secreting PTH autonomously secondary to long-term stimulation.

### 161   A – Addison's disease

This is a rarer cause of hypercalcaemia. Pigmentation of the buccal mucosa and postural hypotension are typical features.

# MANAGEMENT OF BENIGN PROSTATIC HYPERPLASIA

### 162 H – TWOC and $\alpha$-blocker

A recent general anaesthetic and opioid-based analgesia causing constipation are two factors which predispose to developing urinary retention post-operatively. Success rates of TWOC in these circumstances are improved by starting an $\alpha$-blocker 48 hours prior to and after catheter removal.

### 163 D – Open prostatectomy

Symptomatic bladder outflow obstruction secondary to BPH for which medical treatment has failed can be treated by surgery – most commonly TURP or open prostatectomy. Morbidity in patients with large prostates is less if they have an open prostatectomy rather than TURP as this reduces the operation time and avoids excess fluid absorption that can occur during prolonged TURP surgery. Surgery is best avoided in those keen to start a family and remain sexually active due to the risk of impotence.

### 164 B – Finasteride

Finasteride is effective in treating BPH associated with prostates > 30 g and has the additional advantage of reducing prostatic bleeding.

# WOUND COMPLICATIONS

### 165 F – Wound dehiscence

Opening of one or any of the layers of the wound is called dehiscence.

### 166 C – Evisceration

This complete disruption of all the layers of the abdominal wall closure is called evisceration. It is often preceded by a blood-stained watery discharge.

### 167 A – Abscess

The low-grade pyrexia, fullness of the wound and purulent exudate with pressure suggest an abscess is more likely than an infection.

# MANAGEMENT OF HERNIAS

### 168    A – Conservative management

Umbilical hernias in young children should be treated conservatively as most resolve spontaneously. Surgical repair should be reserved for those children in whom the hernia has not resolved by the age of 3 years and the fascial defect is > 1.5 cm in diameter. They should then undergo a repair similar to the 'vest over pants' Mayo repair used for repair of para-umbilical hernias in adults.

### 169    F – Repair via high inguinal (Lotheissen) approach

The Royal College of Surgeons recommends the high inguinal approach for elective repair of femoral hernias, except in thin females where a low crural approach is advised.

### 170    B – Laparoscopic repair

Laparoscopic repair of inguinal hernias is recommended for the management of bilateral inguinal hernias unless there are any contraindications present.

# TREATMENT OF URINARY TRACT INFECTIONS

## 171  G – Rifampicin

Tuberculous urinary infections present with symptoms of recurrent UTIs, weight loss, fever and night sweats. Mid-stream urine shows sterile pyuria. It is usually secondary to renal tuberculosis. It usually responds to anti-tuberculous drugs, but in cases with advanced renal disease, infection may not subside until the involved kidney and ureter have been removed. Diabetic patients are particularly prone to developing UTIs.

## 172  F – Oral ciprofloxacin

If uncomplicated and the patient is systemically well the most common cause is *Escherichia coli* infection and this can be treated with an oral antibiotic such as ciprofloxacin or trimethoprim.

## 173  C – Intravenous co-amoxiclav (Augmentin)

Loin pain, fever and evidence of urine infection should alert to the possibility of ascending infection causing pyelonephritis. Intravenous Augmentin and hospital admission is required.

# POST-OPERATIVE CRITICAL CARE

*Normal values: CVP = 2–8 mmHg; cardiac output = 5 l/min; stroke volume = 60–130 ml*

## 174   C – Hypovolaemic shock

This patient has an increased pulse, decreased CVP, cardiac output and stroke volume, which is consistent with hypovolaemic shock.

## 175   D – Neurogenic shock

The decreased pulse is characteristic of neurogenic shock, which also causes a decreased cardiac output with normal CVP and stroke volume.

## 176   E – Septic shock

The patient has an increased pulse, normal CVP, decreased stroke volume and increased cardiac output, which is consistent with septic shock.

# SKIN LESIONS

**177**  B – Bowen's disease

Full thickness epidermal dysplasia is characteristic of Bowen's disease, which is most common on the lower limbs.

**178**  E – Lentigo maligna

Change in pigmentation is common in lentigo maligna, and 90% of these occur on the face.

**179**  J – Squamous cell carcinoma

Squamous cell carcinoma is most common on sun-exposed areas, frequently bleeds and is characterised by an everted edge.

**180**  A – Basal cell carcinoma

Basal cell carcinoma is characterised by a rolled pearly edge. It does not tend to bleed as often as a squamous cell carcinoma.

# Index

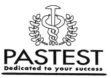